# 21 STEPS TO
# UNSTUCK

You shine! ☆

i

21 STEPS TO UNSTUCK

Copyright © 2023 Dani Simpson

# 21 STEPS TO UNSTUCK

## HOW TO OVERCOME HARD THINGS AND BECOME A HAPPIER, HEALTHIER YOU

I dedicate this book to all the overcomers. May you be empowered, strengthened, equipped and courageously able to transform your minds, live life to the full and positively impact the lives of others. You are world changers; creating ripple effects and tidal waves that shift the course of history for generations to come. May you dynamically transform every sphere of life – from your inner world of wellness to your families, businesses, friendships and relationships.

# 21 STEPS TO UNSTUCK

**A HAPPIER, HEALTHIER YOU!**

**PART 7**
**LET GO AND LAUGH**
Step 19: Adopt an Attitude of Gratitude
Step 20: Forgive Yourself and Others
Step 21: Embrace the Science of Joy and Laughter

**PART 6**
**LIVE – REALLY LIVE**
Step 16: Grow Your Emotional Intelligence (EQ)
Step 17: Find Joy and Value at Work – or Find a New Job!
Step 18: 'Break Up' with Fear Using Journalling

**PART 5**
**STOP LIVING A LIE**
Step 13: Recognise and Resist Your Payoffs
Step 14: Reject Perfectionism
Step 15: Stop Being a False Peacekeeper

**PART 4**
**THE POWER OF MEANINGFUL CONNECTION**
Step 10: Pursue Meaningful Connection
Step 11: Reframe Your Perspective Of Rejection
Step 12: Evaluate, Prune and Grow your Friendships

**PART 3**
**STOP LIVING THE PICTURE IN YOUR HEAD**
Step 7: Set Healthier Boundaries
Step 8: Don't Lose Yourself to Love Someone Else
Step 9: Know the Difference Between your
Core Values and Core Beliefs

**PART 2**
**HAVE BRAVE CONVERSATIONS AND ADDRESS STRESS**
Step 4: Have Braver Conversations with Yourself – Get Real
Step 5: Have Braver Conversations with Others
Step 6: Listen Well – The 'Good Listener' Learns More

**PART 1**
**BREAK THE POWER OF THE WORDS THAT SHAPED YOU**
Step 1: Find Your Own Natural Rhythm, Not Theirs!
Step 2: Remove the 'Sticky Labels' Others Placed on You
Step 3: Break the Limiting Power of Unhelpful Sayings

**START TODAY**

# ABOUT THE AUTHOR

Dani Simpson grew up in Cambridge and Kew Gardens, where her father was a scientist. She had a colourful life and a successful career in sales and marketing before founding a specialist PR business serving London and Surrey for 12 years. Mum of three, Dani grew her passion for wellness in the business sector, initially supporting entrepreneurs. Today she is a successful published author and writer, champions women and supports businesses, schools and charities as a Coach and speaker.

For much of her life, she, like many, battled perfectionism, poor boundaries, people-pleasing, fear, heart pain, trauma and performance-based love, which opened the doors to anxiety, stress and ill health. Dani made it her mission to find freedom, wellness, health, and wholeness. She recognizes the enormity of life's many obstacles, which can often seem overwhelming and insurmountable.

By the grace of God, and with a courageous pursuit for mental and physical wellbeing, Dani overcame chronic health issues, divorce, anxiety, trauma, and depression. She now shares her transformational techniques at Stride Into Life, creating a dynamic modern movement—a tribe for our times—supporting and empowering those who wish to move towards optimal wellness and away from ill health.

## ACCOLADES

Wellness Coach and Author
Founder, Stride Into Life
Health and Wellness Activator, The Great Outdoor Gym Company

Healing and Wholeness Minister, Glasgow Prophetic Centre
Miracle Clinic
NCFE CACHE Level 2 Certification in Domestic Abuse
Founder, The Brand Effect Consultancy
Founder, Market Mall Entrepreneurs
Columnist and Writer
BSc Business Management, Kings College London

# ENDORSEMENTS

Dani is a champion for all who are drawn into her bright and shining orbit. All are impacted by her presence and none will leave it unchanged. Dani's vulnerability offers a beacon of light to all, and allows each one to shine light into their own darkness. The steps in this book are both practical and profound; they will be life-changing for all who courageously choose freedom.

*Sue Jameson,*
*Joy Activist and Laughter Coach,*
*Joyburg, South Africa*

Dani's story results in this very practical and easy to read guide of how to deal with the issues that have and continue to plague our lives. More importantly, this is not a book to be read once and put down. It is one that should be by our side and read continuously to refine how we deal with issues continuously through our lives. It is a book for everyone who wants to deal with hard things; Dani's enthusiasm for wellness and healing is contagious and comes through wonderfully in this journal.

*Dr John Bolodeoku,*
*Consultant Chemical Pathologist and Pharmaceutical Physician,*
*JB Consulting MDP, Berkshire, UK*

There is a saying 'Hurt people, hurt people'. I would like to add that 'Healed people heal people'. Stepping out of the boat may be scary but staying in the boat is devastating – nothing great happens in your comfort zone. If you want to walk on water, you have to get out of the boat! 21 Steps is 21 steps on water. You were created for more so don't settle for less than you were created for. The time for transformation is now. You can make moves, or you can make excuses! If not you, then who? If not now, then when?

*Pastor Raymond Ramos,*
*Recovery House of Worship,*
*New York, USA*

Dani is a trailblazer for anyone looking for the hopeful road to confidence, joy and inner peace. Her 21 Steps will dust you down, clothe you with honour and place a crown upon your head. As a woman, I have drawn tremendous hope and wellbeing from Dani's teachings. I hope you are blessed too, as Dani takes you to the intrinsic and extrinsic promised lands of emotional prosperity, abundance and joy as you apply her transformational steps and techniques.

*Georgina Delaney MBE,*
*CEO The Great Outdoor Gym Company and TGO Activate,*
*Crieff, Scotland*

Dani is an incredible beacon of light. Her holistic emphasis on health and wellbeing is expressed so sensitively – an example to us all.

*Ameenah Ayub- Allen,*
*BAFTA nominated and BIFA-winning Producer, Ali and Ava (2021), Rocks (2019), Brick Lane (2007), London, UK*

I met Dani on 7th November 2019 in Sittingbourne, in a small but charming theatre. What initially struck me was Dani's captivating energy. She filled the room and all of those sitting within it with possibility, confidence, and, most of all, hope for what's to come. Not only was Dani there to learn and find direction for her own ventures, but she was also there to serve, add value and truly support those looking to make positive change.

Over the years, I've watched Dani grow and create incredible things, touching everything around her. I have no doubt that this book will bring you value. Each step will throw you into a headspace you didn't know you had and will aid you in finding the correct path for you in this moment. This book only delivers a fraction of the impact Dani carries and gives to strangers every day. It is truly an honour to know, learn from and work with Dani.

*Henry Nicholson,*
*CEO The Rebel School,*
*London, UK*

Dani is incredibly insightful, and her consistently positive, purposeful and creative personality is an inspiration to me and many others.

*Graham Burns,*
*Chairman, The Change Organisation, Kent, UK*

With incredible insight, positivity and a 'can do' attitude, Dani will no doubt bring out the best in you.

*Professor Michael Bennett OBE,*
*Cambridge, UK*

Dani's genuine empathy and authentic voice in '21 Steps to Unstuck' provides an exceptional companion on the journey of life.

With clarity and passion, Dani imparts invaluable lessons and prompts profound introspection, encouraging readers to embrace their uniqueness and tap into their innate strengths. Whether you're seeking personal fulfilment, professional growth, or a deeper understanding of yourself, '21 Steps to Unstuck' is a must-read and reflects the dynamic programmes and materials developed by Stride Into Life for students and businesses.

Prepare to embark on a transformative journey that will leave you inspired, empowered, and equipped to unleash the extraordinary potential within you. From nurturing self-compassion to cultivating healthy relationships and fostering a resilient mindset, this book is set apart by its comprehensive approach. Dani not only ignites a sense of purpose but also equips readers with the tools necessary to navigate life's challenges with resilience and grace.

*Russell Sauntry,*
*CEO Amelix,*
*Founding Director of Amelix Education,*
*Kent, UK*

# ACKNOWLEDGEMENTS

I am deeply grateful for the countless individuals who have enriched my life and contributed to my journey. My mentor, Tobi, taught me to be a fearless warrior, while Wendy exemplified God's love, belonging, and authentic friendship. Ray guided me towards happiness and health, and Robin unleashed my inner lion, encouraging me to rise in my spheres of influence.

I'm thankful for Jo, who saw past my busyness and connected with my soul, and for Darren, Henry and Paul, who empowered my mind and business. Emma and her team liberated me from paralysis, and Patrick nurtured my love for journaling. Dr. Christian looked beyond my symptoms to provide genuine care, and Restored Lives fortified my heart and mind.

My joy coach, Sue, rekindled my laughter, while Annie and Joanna offered invaluable leadership and direction. I'm forever indebted to my mother, Nina, whose selfless work ethic shaped my character, and my father, Mike, who planted me in Kew to grow and flourish.

Lastly, I extend my heartfelt gratitude to Tony, the pioneer of this book, who bravely illuminated the truths I once denied, ignored, or minimized. His vulnerability and relentless pursuit of truth not only transformed my life but also gave birth to the 21 Steps to Unstuck.

# CONTENTS

# FOREWORD

As you read this, you have in your hands far more than a self-help guide.

First, it comes from the testimony of someone who has lived this out in reality.

Second, it is honest.

Dani does not present herself in these pages as some sort of remote self-help expert but rather a true, sensitive human being, one who knows, who has been there, and who understands our confusion, stress or overwhelm.

At points, you will find yourself thinking, "Dani's like me. If she can do it, I can too."

I find it is all too rare in our culture to find someone who lives by what they say. Here is someone who has lived our pain, who has gone beyond merely "getting by" or survival, but has truly stepped out into a better way of living. Many have given up on that kind of hope.

I have the honour to count Dani a friend and whilst she makes an impact on these pages, I can tell you that she does the same in person. 21 Steps to Unstuck is an authentic expression of who she is: a hope-bringer. And this hope is not merely the fingers-crossed, wishing-as-we-blow-out-birthday-candles kind of fragile hope, but something far, far stronger. This hope amplifies as we go further on that journey with her.

Dani shares her journey from emotional pain and ill health, narrated by all kinds of limiting beliefs commonly shared that she too had believed to be true. That journey led to a very different kind of life, a life of fullness, health, and joy. She says that she is still working that out. She is still growing, still striding. I love that honesty and humility.

Finally, this is a journey beyond the place of, as she puts it, "Not too bad, thanks."

Dani maps out this journey of freedom in these 21 steps, and makes them so accessible to us. She gives us a map, not merely of recovery, but towards a life that we were all meant to live.

This is more than a book about how to get your life and its problems fixed. This is more than curing the dis-ease in your soul or illness in your body. It is more than just getting to "OK". It goes far beyond that.

If you choose, Dani can help you stride into a powerful, positive realm, a life less ordinary.

*Patrick Mayfield, Coach and Author of*
*Leading Yourself; Succeeding from the Inside Out*

# INTRODUCTION

*'Above all else guard your heart....'  Proverb*

If you're reading this book, it is because you feel 'stuck'. Perhaps you have tried everything you can think of to climb out of paralysing fear and worry or move away from your sickness or heart pain. Do friends offer wise advice that worked for 'so and so' but it just doesn't seem to be working for you? Do you wonder how to heal from dis-ease and chronic disease? Do you feel 'wrong inside'? Do you just want to know how to move past the 'debilitating' and towards the 'energising'?

If it's a health or heart by-pass you're after, this book is not for you. But if staying 'stuck' is a worse prospect than facing the hard things keeping you stuck, then keep reading, my friend. You are not alone. Wellness awaits.

I have 21 proven steps that say "YES" to:

- Robust emotional heart surgery (there is no by-pass)

- Dealing with the elephants in the room

- Challenging and changing unhelpful beliefs and assumptions

- Reframing what happened

- Optimal wellness (physical and emotional)

- Stepping out of fear and pain

- Moving forwards in your relationships, career and life

Thank you for allowing me walk with you on this part of your journey. We'll face some tough stuff together, but we'll find the way out.

There is a way out.

Will it be easy? Nope. Can you do it? Absolutely!

## BREAK THROUGH

In Michael Rosen's book 'We're going on a Bear Hunt,' the family face challenges but recognise "We can't go over it, we can't go under it, we can't go round it. We'll have to go through it". And they do!

In the real world, we try not to 'go through it' but instead find reasons to hide from, deny or ignore 'it'. However, this approach can cause emotional trauma and chronic disease.

So, let's do something better. Let's 'go through it'. Together.

For me, the sensation of knowing I was ready to face my fears, pain and stuckness felt much like standing in the eye of a tornado—quiet, still, kind of eerie, and unnerving. Yet, there was a tingle of anticipation that I would finally 'do this' and get 'through it,' emerging into the sunshine.

Hold onto that tingle. It may feel tiny but rest assured it's enough.

When you feel like a grape going through a 'crushing' process, confronting the crushing things you've been avoiding (or ignoring) can create something wonderful.

Crushed grapes become champagne.

This verse someone shared with me was truly helpful, too "A bruised reed He (God) will not break [off] and a dimly burning wick He will not extinguish; He will faithfully bring forth justice...' from Isaiah 42 in the Bible. It provided me with a) a broader perspective and b) the reassurance to trust God to help me on the journey. Let's be honest, most of us fear that if we dare to delve deep into our inner world or confront the obstacles keeping us stuck in life, we might 'break.'

## WHY CAN'T WE STAY IN THE PIT OF GRIEF, STRESS, PAIN, FEAR OR DYSFUNCTION?

The feeling of dis-ease caused by staying stuck for too long causes disease.

For me, this meant being diagnosed with depression, myalgic encephalomyelitis (ME), fibromyalgia, chronic eczema, urticaria, endocrine dysfunction, and post-traumatic stress disorder (PTSD). In simpler terms, fear, heartache, and mental, emotional, or spiritual distress can manifest as illness and physical aches and pains. For you, maybe its headaches, back pain or something else. It's no way to live. This state of being creates lifelessness.

So, allow me to clarify what I mean by 'staying' in a place of pain or dysfunction.

'Staying' means:

1) doing nothing.

2) repeating the same cycles over and again, hoping for different results.

3) rushing around in a failed attempt numb the pain.

4) running away.

For me, the most disabling symptom of 'staying' in the place of dysfunction was chronic fatigue and problems with thinking and memory. At one point, I asked my GP if she could test me for dementia, but she assured me it was simply stress manifesting itself.

The body reacts to the environment it is in, and so I discovered that the trauma and exhaustion present in my environment needed to be confronted, not ignored. If I was created for wellness (which entails much more than just the absence of disease), then I could take steps toward wellness without fearing that I would break along the way. I was not broken; I was merely displaying symptoms of chronic stress and turmoil.

You are not broken; you are whole; your body has mental and physical health within it and an innate ability to heal. You were created for wellness and wholeness, for love and life.

So staying in the place of dysfunction doesn't work for us. We need to do something......

**GO 'ROUND IT?' NO**

When we avoid pain, we can end up going around in circles with no clear solutions in sight.

# INTRODUCTION

We've walked around this mountain too many times!

We've denied, ignored, and minimised what we're afraid to confront for long enough now!

We've shied away from taking responsibility for the things we'd rather run away from!

We discovered that our survival tactics don't work very well for us!

## GLOSS OVER IT? NOPE...

When we minimise our inner world of feeling shut down, devoid of hope or in fear, it's not a nurturing or nourishing place to be. We need nourishment. We need nurturing. We need to live. Really live.

We were not born to live masked by smiles, busyness, unhealthy habits, denial or addictions to drink, food, workaholism, self-centredness, porn or dare I say, even religion. By this, I mean a regimented adherence to rules and regulations as a coping tool, as opposed to a helpful and meaningful spiritual relationship with God.

You were not born to live 'stressed' or 'distressed'. You were created to live in peace and wellness.

## GO THROUGH IT? YES!

When we find and face discomfort and difficult things, we find emotional wellness, physical health and freedom.

Would you go about your day with grit in your eye, knowing it would cause damage if left there? Unlikely. Your eyes matter. So, you'd dislodge it even if it hurt. And you'd heal.

So why go about your day with niggly grit in your heart or mind – the sources of life itself? Your heart and mind matter. You matter. So, it's time to dislodge it. Even if it hurts, you'll heal.

I'm not trying to get you from A-Z. But I do hope to help you move at least some way towards your emotional freedom and physical healing.

4

As we journey, remember I'm in my own lane and you are in yours. I won't tell you *what* to think, but rather *how* to think through 21 common barriers to find the root(s) of being stuck and build the resilience to move forwards. There are just 7 parts to navigate.

**BUT, YOU SAY, YOU DON'T KNOW WHAT HAPPENED TO ME!**

I don't know what happened and I'm sorry it happened to you. I'm sorry about what they did. I'm sorry that many of the seemingly unscalable walls are not your fault — faulty teaching, neglect, misunderstanding, abuse, pain, stress, betrayal or mistakes...

Let's move away from that pain now and take 21 steps towards a happier, healthier you.

# INTRODUCTION

# PART 1
# BREAK THE POWER OF THE WORDS
# THAT SHAPED YOU

Words are a creative force, so the first three steps will show you how to come unstuck from the words that have kept you down

# STEP 1: FIND YOUR OWN RYTHYM

# STEP 1: Find Your Own Natural Rhythm, Not Theirs!

Identify who you've emulated and give them back their own lane.

*'Comparison is the thief of joy'*
*- T. Roosevelt*

## HELEN

*Helen tried to keep up with Sam as she wound her way to the theatre bar. Sam's life always seemed so full-on. Glancing at the ice creams and gourmet popcorn, Helen's mind wandered away from the West End to Sam's many tech companies and interests. Dad would have been so proud of her. She seemed to be everything he'd wanted in a daughter.*

*Didn't Sam ever get tired? How did she cram so much into a day? Sam fired off emails and created reels while they waited in line.*

> *"Make every second count sis," said Sam." You'll be spinning more plates than me one day".*

*Helen ignored the discomfort she felt.  Life would feel less overwhelming soon, surely. The stillness of her studio in St Albans felt wonderful, but she reasoned she'd better join the family business in London before too long. Her sister laughed as someone called her name.*

# STEP 1: FIND YOUR OWN RYTHYM

**H**urry up! Come on, slow, coach! Can't you go any faster? So often, we feel out of sorts because we are living life at a speed that feels unnatural to us. Often, our learned behaviours, habits and rhythms are natural to the people around us but feel unnatural to us – yet we do them anyway.  Why?

A       We were quite simply raised at that pace, and it went unquestioned by us whether that pace of life is beneficial to us or causes discomfort and dis-ease.

or

B       We know the pace isn't right, but we want the money, status or other payoffs the pace brings – even if it is hurting us.

For this step, I'm talking mostly to readers in camp A who don't know they are living outside of their natural rhythm.

Are you emulating someone else's rhythm? Are you sick and tired of feeling sick and tired, stressed, frustrated, de-energised or just not quite right?

Tell-tale signs that you may be living by someone else's rhythm, not your own.

- Low energy
- Feeling out of sorts or out of alignment
- Overwhelmed
- A sense of dis-ease
- Feeling not enough or unable to keep up the pace (too slow or too fast)
- Underlying frustration
- Feeling stressed
- Physical symptoms – like unsettled sleep or skin conditions

## STEP 1: FIND YOUR OWN RYTHYM

Your natural rhythm is *not* the pace unwittingly set for you by parents or caregivers many years ago. It is the natural pace of life for you. And it's important you find it.

Parents and caregivers didn't set your rhythm of life on purpose – (they respond to environmental stimuli and circumstances, and create their own rhythms) – but nevertheless, they do set your pace.

Now though, you are empowered to re-calibrate your rhythm and live your authentic life – at your own pace.

**WHAT IS YOUR NATURAL RHYTHM?**

I lived for years, out of sync and out of sorts. As a child, we lived between two houses—our family home in Cambridge and our rental house in Kew, near my father's laboratory. As you can imagine, life was busy for Mum— working full time, looking after two homes, raising three children, caring for the wider family, and doing voluntary work. Dad was a scientist and worked long hours, in addition to writing books and lecturing.

I remember my Nannie exclaiming, 'Wow, your mum doesn't walk; she runs!'. So mostly, we ran too.

Our shopping trips to town on weekends were something akin to 'Challenge Anneka'. We raced round the supermarket doing our weekly shop like an episode of 'Supermarket Sweep'.

It was all normal. It was just 'life'.

As a result, my go-to speed was set to fast. So, for me, if I couldn't keep up, I felt like I'd just have to do better and go faster.

The discomfort and feelings of overwhelm I had inside felt normal to me, but my body was telling me I needed time to realign my rhythm of life. At 16, I was put on beta blockers for so-called anxiety. It wasn't until years later I realised I wasn't naturally anxious; I was quite simply living a pace of life that was unnatural for me – the weekly 200-mile commute, living in the public eye in Kew Gardens, leading youth work, pursuing fitness, managing school work, volunteering, tending two gardens...

I sat down one day to ask myself, what is my natural pace? I'm a writer. A deep thinker. A speaker. An empath. A mentor. A coach. A person who needs time to process thoughts, feelings, and ideas. I enjoy taking time to crystalise concepts, inhabit creative spaces and get into a zone that allows creative juices to flow. And that's okay.

What was mum's natural pace? A PA for many years, mum's job suited her natural aptitude for speedy organisation, practicality, caring for the people and places around her and juggling many jobs at once. I'm in awe how she got so much done in a day – volunteer work, gardening, housekeeping, hosting, and a full-time job. Her pace was phenomenal. Her pace was okay for her.

What was Dad's natural pace? Dad was a Professor, Fellow and scientist who took time to study and write many books and scientific papers, spending long hours 'on task', managing teams and overseeing phenomenally large budgets for projects of global significance. His capacity and ability earned him an OBE. His pace was okay for him.

But both unknowingly set high bench marks I felt unable to attain – in terms of my speed or accolades. I always felt incapable of going fast enough and beat myself up that my straight As were not A* or A**. Comparison raised its ugly head for years until one day, I realised that I could operate well at my own natural rhythm. I just had to find it.

## HOW TO FIND YOUR NATURAL RHYTHM

- Do you like quiet time to work at your optimal level?
- Are you energised when you're busy and when you're at home, or when you're out?
- Does it frustrate or satisfy you to do things slowly and methodically?

13

- Are you overtired or buzzing when you complete your to-do list speedily?
- Do you find joy and ease in multitasking, or do you prefer to focus on one task at a time?
- Are you analytical or expressive?

I used to feel guilty about taking time to pause or think deeply about ideas, concepts, editorials or coaching. I used to sense discomfort when planning how I'll take ideas and translate them into digestible articles, content, and courses. I don't anymore.

I learned it's just how I'm wired.

It sometimes means I forget to do other things, get into the zone and arrive late at social dates. I'm working on it but give myself grace when it happens.

Sometimes when I'm quiet – I'm thinking. People ask me if I'm okay or if I'm happy. I am so happy. I'm just processing while I'm meandering, exercising, taking a walk or doing a stretch class. I need time to chew on things. By the end of a walk or gym session, I have crystalised the vision, know how to reach the goal and can get on with the day.

How about you? Will you choose to take Step 1 and move away from feeling uncomfortable about your failure to operate in the same way as so and so? You were never meant to. That rhythm doesn't fit you.

You are free to align with your own natural pace and finding your own rhythm is an ongoing exercise.

The most significant initial hurdle here is admitting that you've been emulating someone else's natural pace and suffering because of it. However, this realisation is not a failure; it's a win. You don't need to hurry up or slow down! You get to be kind to yourself and find your own balance.

Well, done for noticing things are out of sync. Well done for spotting the dis-ease. Now you can choose to redress the imbalance, reflect on how you are wired and live more authentically. Catch yourself this week when you feel out of sync, and realign yourself with your own natural rhythm. Set sensible time scales to complete tasks. Give yourself the time you need to walk, work, socialise, commute, think, reflect, and live.

**REFLECTING ON THIS STATEMENT CAN BE HELPFUL**

As a child, I learned what life looks like and figured out how to adapt to fit in with my environment and family. But as an adult, I need to take time to identify when I am living in ways that are not a good fit for me. I choose to explore my authentic self and be true to myself, not to live at the speed modelled to me by parents or caregivers. I can set the pace that's right for me. I can find my balance, and if I get it wrong, I can always recalibrate.

What is your natural rhythm?

_____
_____
_____
_____
_____
_____
_____
_____
_____

# STEP 1: FIND YOUR OWN RYTHYM

## STEP 2: Remove the Sticky Labels Others Placed on You

Reclaim your authentic self by taking back your power from the people who labelled you in life

*'As you think, so shall you become.'*
- Bruce Lee

**RUBY**

*Ruby shrieked with delight as her plaits dangled on the daisies in the long grass. She had finally mastered headstands. When she wasn't practicing, she would sit in the treehouse shouting down to the neighbours who passed along the garden wall.*

> *"Hi Diana," she said, waving animatedly as Tom came round the corner.*

> *"Oh wow, that's a huge bag Tom; what did you buy?". But before Tom could even reply, she had spotted Mrs Elma gardening and jumped up to see what she was pruning.*

> *"Hey, Mrs Elma, did you see me with my new baby cousin last week? She's so tiny. I love your new red roses!".*

*Mum had been especially quiet the last few weeks and as the back door opened, Ruby knew what was coming.*

> *"Get down from there and come inside. You're so loud, Ruby. The neighbours don't want you bothering them," scolded mum.*

*Ruby sloped into the breakfast bar. Her school report had said she's 'gregarious', but mum seemed much happier when Ruby was quiet.*

# STEP 2: REMOVE STICKY LABELS

Who we believe we are determines our state of wellbeing. Winner or loser. Valued or worthless. Weak or strong. Shy or assertive.

Every day we ask others 'How are you?' but we rarely ask the question that matters most, 'Who are you?'.

'Who are you?' is the most important question of all. It's the question we need to keep asking ourselves to get free from the sticky labels others placed on us; the shy one, the sickly one....

As everything in life starts with a thought or belief (which then creates an action), it's fundamental to know if you are living as your true authentic self *or* if you are living a projected version of yourself.

This 'self' is projected onto us (knowingly or unknowingly) by caregivers, culture, society, friendship groups and learned behaviours. It serves whoever placed the sticky labels on us very well and they likely had no idea of the impact of doing so. An example might be a quiet parent who feels shy and overwhelmed, labelling their child as domineering, loud and bossy. But really? Are they? Or does the parent simply feel intimidated by the child's gregarious nature?

This, of course, becomes more complex when dealing with abuse, where mean language is used to label, name-call, and control—but we'll address that in Step 8. Step 2 is to reclaim your power and recentre yourself.

**WHO TOOK THE POWER IN THE FIRST PLACE?**

Powerful people in your life include your parents, your boss, your spouse, your partner, friends, peers, the media, the movie industry, the culture you grew up in...

Perhaps you've been made to feel like or been labelled as....

- The loud child
- The smart daughter
- The bossy one
- The emotional wreck

- The easy (or accommodating) child
- The difficult one

Did those labels ever really fit you back then?

Do they fit you now?

As you read this chapter, begin thinking about the labels you've acquired. Take time to notice and reflect on them, and we'll do an exercise to remove those which are incorrect or no longer accurate later in this chapter.

Reclaiming your identity is the foundation of all the other steps.

Sign your name here as you begin to consider and reflect on who you are.

**Name:**

_____

## ADAPT TO FIT

As a child, you learned quickly how to 'adapt to fit' with carers' needs and expectations, their ideologies and their feelings about you and your role. It's quite simply a human condition, but we no longer need to 'play out what they say out'.

*'We no longer need to play out what they say out'* - Raymond Ramos

Raymond's words are wise and especially true if those labels were or are derogatory – annoying, stupid, irritant, boring, clumsy or deceitful. They apply in the case of more generic labels, too; shy, sickly, bossy or messy...

Most of us are unaware of the intensely powerful impact of words and labels. But we no longer need to stay stuck playing out the roles or labels assigned to us.

### "YOU'RE TOO TALL!"

Much of the time, the way people label you in life, says more about their own perceived inadequacies than it does about you.

The person who called you 'too tall' was likely intimidated by your height or self-conscious about theirs.

The person who called you 'bossy' or 'loudmouth' may have felt degrees of discomfort and inferiority around your outgoing personality compared to their more reserved nature.

The person who labelled you 'stupid' or 'too much' likely suffered low esteem or plain old frustration in the moment, and lacked patience or self-control. It was never about 'you'.

### NAMES WILL NEVER HURT ME. NONSENSE!

Were you ever called a name at school, and it stuck in your sub-conscious?

Were you labelled by your boss and so lost confidence?

Were you belittled or called 'idiot' by someone?

The saying 'sticks and stones may break my bones, but names will never hurt me' is simply not true. Names and labels can hurt a lot and become debilitating if we let them.

We carry labels which have defined us and which we believe are okay or even true of us. Often, they are not true at all!

**WHAT IS NORMAL AND WHAT IS TRUE?**

As mental health awareness grows, we are rightly encouraged to seek help when we need it and the first thing my counsellor did when I was struggling myself was to help me question what I believed was normal, true or acceptable.

Whatever you've been labelled – in childhood, relationships or work – it may have served you well to play the role you were assigned (for protection or to navigate your environment the best you knew how), but there's no longer a requirement to live a projected version of yourself. A happier and healthier you awaits your "Yes".

Along with all the labels we carry, there tends to be a go-to label that feels bigger than all the rest. Mine was 'Be seen and not heard'. What is yours? Is it true? Write your go-to label here and begin to question if it's true. Who gave it to you? Why might they have done that?

My go-to label:

_____

**FROM WOUNDS TO WELLNESS**

Humans desire wellness, healing and happiness, but waiting for circumstances to align and heal our soul wounds elongates the healing process and the journey towards these priceless things.

So rather than wait for circumstances to align, if we instead transform our minds, thoughts and feelings, we can choose freedom from the power of unhelpful words. And from that place, we can create the life we desire to lead.

**FREEDOM IN OUR INNER WORLD CREATES FREEDOM IN OUR OUTER WORLD**

As human beings, we *all* have common fears; we are afraid of failure. Of rejection. Of being 'not enough. Or of being 'too much'.

You are 'enough' and you have all you need to love yourself well.

You can walk into wellness as a matter of choice *not* because you feel like it. As you do this, you begin to partner with what you are wired for – truth, hope, positivity, and love.

I lived for years believing I couldn't do public speaking and should be seen but not heard. However, I chose to reclaim my authentic self and challenge my limiting beliefs. As a first step, I trained staff at workshops in London; then I chaired meetings with prospective marketing clients. I built on this by leading kid's teams at my local church and a significant milestone in my breaking free was speaking at a women's conference the day after my father-in-law died.

I replaced 'I can't do public speaking' with 'I can do this'. Although I was nervous, and still am sometimes, I did it. You can too! What will be your first practical step to challenge and disprove the 'go-to' label assigned to you and the limiting belief it created? Note that down here.

---

One day, the fear of staying stuck becomes greater than the fear of stepping out. Your breakthrough day is today, and every day.

**SEEN AND NOT HEARD**

The saying 'children should be seen and not heard' has caused generations of children and adults to remain stuck.

If this is you, too, I apologise on behalf of whoever said it to you.

You were born to be seen and heard.

You can find your voice, and I can too. As adults, parents, bosses, friends, and neighbours, we need to understand this truth: "me finding my voice doesn't diminish you finding yours. There's room in this world for all of us."

---

Me finding my voice doesn't diminish you finding yours. There's room in this world for all of us.

---

Thankfully the world has moved on from the Mary Poppins era of parenting, where children were kept quiet and out of sight. Today emotional health forms part of their curriculum, mental health week is championed, children follow programmes like Heart Smart and charities promote awareness campaigns, and initiatives like anti-bullying week.

## BE TRUE TO YOURSELF

Roleplaying is mentally, emotionally, and physically exhausting. And may be making you unwell (tired, stressed, anxious, depressed). You are free to be yourself no matter who you are with.

The easiest way to figure out who you truly are is to reflect on how you carry yourself with different groups of people in your life. Are you the same 'you' in different settings? When are you playing a role versus feeling comfortable, natural and confident?

Pick your favourite and your least favourite colour. Circle the words that are authentically you in your favourite colour, then circle all the words that have been projected into you or spoken over you (by yourself or others) in the other colour. Some labels may have 2 colours and that's ok.

Add your own words and characteristics too. What words (limiting thoughts or beliefs) have you had or heard about yourself that are not who you really are?

NICE MEAN BRIGHT CHEERFUL CARING BOLD CONSIDERATE EMOTIONAL KIND PEACEFUL PLEASANT POLITE PEOPLE-PLEASER SWEET THOUGHTFUL COOPERATIVE LONER ACTIVE NON-COOPERATIVE CALM STRESSED DEPENDABLE IRRESPONSIBLE HUMBLE PROUD IMMATURE MATURE PATIENT ANGRY UNKIND RUDE UNTRUSTWORTHY UNDEPENDABLE DISHONEST CONCEITED IMPATIENT DOWN ANXIOUS BRAVE ASSERTIVE BOSSY CERTAIN UNCERTAIN LOSER STUPID FUNNY GENTLE CLOWN GLAMOROUS BIG-HEADED SHY QUIET HYPER SERIOUS SIMPLE LOUD SLOW NOISY ROUGH UNATTRACTIVE FLIRTY BORING AMBITIOUS ADVENTUROUS BRASSY BUSY HARD-WORKING BOFFIN NERD GEEK DULL INDIFFERENT LAZY NEGLECTFUL SLUGGISH UNREALISTIC INEXPERIENCED COURAGEOUS FEARLESS FEARFUL INDEPENDENT SURE HESITANT ANXIOUS UNEASY SELF-CONSCIOUS UNFAIR MEEK ANTISOCIAL GLOOMY GLUM COMFORTLESS EMPATH DEPRESSIVE GLUM NERVOUS HEARTBREAKER HEARTBROKEN HOPELESS HELPLESS MISERABLE MOODY WITHDRAWN UNHAPPY CRUEL EVIL HATEFUL RUDE UNFRIENDLY UNCARING DARK DISRESPECTFUL HARSH UGLY NOTHING IMPOLITE SPOILED THOUGHTLESS STRESSFUL

_____
_____
_____
_____
_____
_____
_____
_____
_____
_____

Having completed this exercise, write a letter telling yourself you are enough. This can be emotionally challenging if we have spent our life being told or believing we are not enough, so be kind to yourself and come back to this any time. I've written an example for inspiration:

*Dear Not Enough*

I am enough!

I can't be smaller because you are offended by my bigness. I can't shine less because you are put off by my brightness. I won't keep quiet because you don't approve of what I have to say. I won't shape shift to become the definition of what makes you feel comfortable. I won't fail to take up the space given to me because you'd rather I didn't.

I won't stop building because you want me stuck in the mud. I won't stop equipping myself because you are threatened by my knowledge or understanding. I won't stop walking into my destiny because you are not happy for me. I won't let my successful outcome be limited by your jealousy.

I won't let your lane become my lane, or your dream become my dream. I have gifts and talents unique to me. I won't belittle them in order to make you feel better about yourself.

I am loved and loveable. I was made to be authentically 'me' so I daily find and peel off the sticky labels others stuck on me that don't 'fit'.

I choose not to emulate anyone – their characteristics or their life. I am open to being honest with myself. So I choose to notice what has made me feel unworthy, inadequate, wrong or embarrassed and peel off every label that doesn't fit me. I retain the ones that do.

I choose to keep – kind, joyful, intelligent, tall, optimistic, gregarious, creative and courageous. I choose to live as the very best version of myself. I don't need to entertain thoughts of comparison, low self-esteem, fear, rejection, dis-ease, shame or embarrassment any longer and if people have told me I am not enough, they are wrong.

I am free to occupy my space. And you yours. There is enough space for everyone.

I am enough!

*All the best, Dani x*

# STEP 3: Break the Limiting Power of Unhelpful Sayings
## Create an atmosphere conducive to health and happiness

*'This day is going from bad to worse'*
- Someone you know

**DAVE**

*Dave was already bracing himself for his parents' criticism.*

> *"You should be ashamed of yourself Dave; come on. After 25 years, you might have remembered your brother's birthday," said mum.*

*Dave felt bad and shrank back into his seat. He'd had a lot on his plate recently with the leaky roof, overseas projects and conferences. Sleep was scarce and his daughter was teething.*

*He'd posted the gift? At least, he thought he had.*

> *"This day is going from bad to worse son," Mum continued. "I smashed a glass, your brother is upset and we all know bad things come in threes, so what next? And where are you anyway, love? If you're driving to London again, you'll never get parking. Sod's Law you'll get a ticket too, just like Becky did".*

# STEP 3: BREAK THE LIMITING POWER

A good life is rooted in a healthy thought life, so for Step 3 we need to find and catch our thoughts that are quite frankly untrue. They cause us to live in negativity, expecting the worst and they've become part of the fabric of our life.

Bad things come in threes. Really?!

A good thought life not only prevents brain damage but positively impacts our all-round health. Negative thoughts and habitual negative phrases are like little foxes. They often go unquestioned or unnoticed but create many dark tunnels in our minds.

**TRANSFORM YOUR MIND**

To retake a driving test after years of driving, most of us would have to unlearn bad habits picked up along the way. It's the same principle in life. We need to unlearn some of the unhealthy ways our minds work and then create more positive ways of thinking.

Healthier thoughts produce healthier emotions, which produce healthier actions, so we start at the beginning with our minds.

We owe it to ourselves to do an audit of the words we think and speak because words have power. We can change the sayings, words and phrases we use that are unhelpful and de-energising, both for us and those around us. According to Carolyn St John Loder, Chief Executive of Health Coaches Academy, it takes 36 weeks to cement a new habit. That includes 3 weeks to break it, 6 weeks to establish a new one and 36 weeks for it to become the new normal or default way of thinking.

Transforming the mind is a two-part process. The first part is to stop voicing the negative or limiting statement, and the second is to replace it with a more positive and uplifting truth.

Let's be real, we've all lived, and life comes with challenges which cause us feelings of overwhelm, stress, dis-ease, worry and fear. But no matter the circumstances, you can embrace deeper levels of wellbeing by thinking about what you're thinking about – more carefully!

**STOP YOUR DAY GOING FROM BAD TO WORSE**

So, do words *really* have a significant impact have on our bodies, feelings and actions? Let's see;

Imagine you're sitting on the beach on a hot summer's day, watching an air show overhead. Your friend is swimming in the sea just in front of you. You can smell the sea, taste the sea air, see the crowds and hear children shrieking with delight. All is well, but suddenly a plane falls out of the sky and crashes just a few feet in front of you. You can't see your friend. The plane is inverted and the pilot is trapped under the waves in the cockpit.

How do you feel now? This incident is not happening – it's just words - but you are having a physical reaction to them. Thankfully this pilot escaped with minor injuries and my friend was fine too.

**OUR MINDS ARE POWERFUL**

Thoughts (disbelief and shock) create feelings (fear) and actions (racing heart, churning stomach, eyes wide, gasps or shortness of breath).

Words are a creative force that shifts atmospheres.

So, if I say, 'my day is going to bad to worse,' I have created a statement that creates my own reality and consequently that of those around me who are brought into my negative atmosphere.

It's clear that society is sick with this dis-ease so there's a pressing need to:

- Renew our thinking
- Reframe our feelings
- Realign our actions

**30,000 THOUGHTS A DAY**

Communication pathologist and cognitive neuroscientist Dr Caroline Leaf shares how 75% to 95% of illnesses are a direct result of our thought life. We have 30,000 thoughts a day, and 80% of these are negative, so when we don't take control of our minds, the damage to our physical and emotional health is significant. We are fuelling an epidemic of negativity and toxicity.

The situation is made worse, of course, by people intentionally using words to confuse, manipulate, or hurt others. We see this happening more frequently as the incidences of stress, addiction, and domestic abuse rise year after year. It's sobering that domestic abuse cases now account for 14.1% of all court prosecutions, and in 2022, the volume rose to the highest level ever (The Crime Survey for England and Wales CSEW, ending March 2022).

The truth is, we can't control what happens in life, but we *can* protect our mental health by training ourselves to respond to our thoughts and words in healthier ways, limit stress and prevent angry red mist from rising

As a society, we are fostering sickness and stress by trusting the negative and unhelpful phrases we use, as well as the atmospheres they create. Our minds are sick with negativity. We have accepted so much of it as normal. However, the truth is that there is no such thing as Sod's law, and bad things don't come in threes.

We have a choice about what we're thinking and saying. I used to believe que sera sera (what will be will be) – and so it was. I lived disempowered, believing I had little or no control over my destiny and sure enough, I then had no control over the day.

**EXAMPLE**

**A Que Sera Sera Day**

Woke up late, missed the train, chronic fatigue, got to work late, itchy eczema, late for staff meeting, tasteless lunch in the staff canteen, fibromyalgia pains, drove the temperamental fleet car for afternoon appointments, out for departmental drinks, went home via the supermarket, made pasta, fire-fighting paperwork, flicked through television channels, landed on an average documentary, fell asleep on the sofa.

However, now I know I don't need to accept 'what is' but can take steps to change it, so the same day goes like this.

**Versus an Empowered Day**

Woke up early, prepared a salad, did Pilates, journaled, felt energised, caught the train to work, contacted the editorial team, pre-booked the new fleet car, excelled in the staff meeting, enjoyed homemade salad for lunch, breezed through afternoon appointments, went out for drinks with the editorial team, headed home via the supermarket, made fresh pasta, filed papers, enjoyed a film I wanted to see, engaged in meditative prayers, and went to bed on time.

## THE PROGRESSION TO DEPRESSION

Negative speaking and thinking are part of the progression to stress and depression, so as a society, we are not helping ourselves with the de-energising and unhelpful things we say.

Rather than deny, minimise, and ignore the words in our environment that cause dis-ease, it's wise to find and uproot them to turn the tide and reduce stress responses, physical disease and lasting mental health issues. Words and sayings can be so harmful to our health!

## WHAT ARE YOU THINKING!?

What words, sayings, phrases and faulty thinking/negative beliefs or ideologies have you brought into your adult life and relationships?

Which sayings do you commonly use, and how do they negatively impact your thoughts, wellbeing, and actions?

Add your own to my list and you may also find it helpful to imagine these negative toxic words are a toxic drink or meal. They can all be replaced with helpful energising alternatives. Which would you prefer to consume? A toxic beverage or an energy drink?

| Unhelpful, de-energising go-to thoughts, words and phrases | Can be replaced with helpful, energising go-to thoughts, words and phrases |
|---|---|
| Que Sera, Sera, whatever will be will be | I'm going to focus on life-giving positive thoughts and words because I am not disempowered. I have the creative power to shape my day with joy, love and happiness. |
| This will all end in tears | The kids are having so much fun...I'll laugh with them, or join in! |
| Sod's Law: It's going to go wrong! | That was tough but things will surely get better |
| It never rains but it pours | This is challenging but grows my character and makes me stronger |
| Fake it til you make it | I know who I am and I love being authentically me. No-one is perfect and I give myself the freedom to fail sometimes. I learn from my mistakes |
| This day is going from bad to worse | Tomorrow will be a better day |
| Ignorance is bliss | Knowledge is power. I am empowered when I face hard things and confront them. |
| Cor Blimey! (God blind me) | Wow!! |

| | |
|---|---|
| You should be ashamed of yourself! | I forgive you and release myself |
| This is Impossible! | There's a way forward, even if I don't know it yet. |
| Bad things happen in threes | What happened wasn't great but it doesn't determine what happens next. |
| Kill them with kindness | My emotional tank is empty, so I need to be kind to 'me' |

*Add your own....*

| | |
|---|---|
| _____ | _____ |
| _____ | _____ |
| _____ | _____ |
| _____ | _____ |

It's important to remember Step 3 is both reactive and proactive. The reactive part is taking negative thoughts captive and choosing to stop saying them. The proactive part replaces unhelpful thoughts, words and phrases with more energising healthy alternatives.

## HOW HAVE NEGATIVE BELIEFS AND SPEECH IMPACTED MY EVERY DAY?

Negative thinking creates hopelessness, helplessness and inaction. When I use negative words and phrases, I communicate to myself and those around me that....

I expect the worst...

I fail to confront things...

I feel like the day will get worse so I project that atmosphere...

I see tears, not joy, on the horizon...

I stop my kids goofing around...

I live in a victim state...

I expect my health to deteriorate....

My hope levels are low...

I feel stressed and not much like laughing....

I complain a lot....

## HOW DO POSITIVE BELIEFS AND WORDS IMPACT MY DAY?

I'm hopeful and trust things will get better

I feel more light-hearted and less stressed

I face problems and seek solutions

I project confidence

I confront hard things

I allow myself to wallow for a while, but I don't stay there for too long

I reframe rather than complain

I understand that depression is a progression

I notice my body's warning signals rather than ignoring them

## STEP 3: BREAK THE LIMITING POWER

I shift negative atmospheres

I lead the way, irrespective of my job title

I am a powerful force for change and for good

**DON'T HURT ME!**

'Blimey' (blind me) is an interesting phrase. It's so commonplace so we've come to accept it as normal. But I propose it's far from normal to say 'Harm me, dis-able me, blind me or hurt me' when we can replace 'blimey' with awe and wonder, 'Wow!'.

The key to breakthrough in Step 3 is to move towards a way of thinking, speaking and being that is whole and undivided.

In Step 3, we choose to be proactively positive in thought and action. We walk the walk. And talk the talk. What we do and say adds up. We don't leak negativity and begin to radiate positivity and wellness.

When mind, body and spirit are in sync in your life, you'll experience more energy and vitality (yes, please!).

Reflect and build your awareness daily. As you do this step, you'll create new neural pathways, which become new superhighways of go-to thinking.

In her book Switch on Your Brain, Dr Caroline Leaf explains how moment by moment, every day, you are changing the structure of your brain through your thinking. When captured visually in scientific testing, Dr Leaf found that healthy thoughts look like spongey trees that attract more healthy thoughts, and unhealthy thoughts look like gnarly toxic trees that attract more of the same.

Science invites us to build healthy forests of good thought trees in our minds.

Step 3, like many of the other steps, is an ongoing process, and this is exciting because whilst catching your own thoughts, words and phrases, you can also help others catch theirs.

## PART 1 ACTIVATIONS

## PAY IT FORWARD - EMPOWER OTHERS

**Step 1:**

Release your family or anyone else you need to from trying to emulate your natural rhythm and encourage them to find and follow their own

**Step 2:**

Contact the people you have labelled and release them from the labels you gave them, explaining what you have learned about the power of sticky labels

**Step 3:**

Create happier, healthier families and friendships by helping others catch unhelpful phrases and bring positive changes to our lives

# STEP 3: BREAK THE LIMITING POWER

# PART 2
# HAVE BRAVE CONVERSATIONS AND ADDRESS STRESS

Denying, ignoring and minimising hard things is unhelpful, so the next
three steps will empower you to have braver conversations with yourself
and others. You will discover how to alleviate stress by confronting
issues and clearing elephants in the room

# STEP 3: BREAK THE LIMITING POWER

# STEP 4: Have Braver Conversations with Yourself – Get Real

## Reduce the stress you are experiencing

*'45% of people suffer from long term chronic stress and more experience acute stress regularly'*
*- Patrick Holford*

## PETE

*Pete had been called a sissy by his father. His sisters were so-called drama queens. He'd begun to notice how much happier his father was when he didn't express how he was truly feeling.*

*Gradually he was unable to express himself at all.*

*As he walked along platform 3, he became aware of a silent scream inside. It had been taunting him in recent months and seemed to be getting louder. He really disliked it. He'd be fine soon.*

*He noticed some people near him being goofy with each other and a teenage girl being bear-hugged by her dad. His stomach tightened. He had no time to goof around or cry; he had an important job. When you're a CEO, feelings are just a nuisance aren't they? He felt a tug on his heart. To make it stop he played a podcast and searched LinkedIn. His network was vast.*

# STEP 4: HAVE BRAVER CONVERSATIONS WITH YOURSELF

Let's be honest; most of us are scared of ourselves. We're scared about our embarrassing or shameful feelings, our fears, our heart pain, our perceived inadequacies, and our poor reactions to things. However, being more transparent about these things removes much of the stress associated with them.

Rather than take a scary dive into our inner world, we have mostly run away from ourselves. Step 4 is to stop running away from yourself and courageously confront hard things to help prevent unwanted stress in your life. So many of us dislike confrontation, but confronting hard things is healthy and the more we do it, the easier it becomes. It may help to replace 'confront' with 'carefront' because your care is a positive quality.

**HEALTH WARNING**

This is not the most pleasant process (the truth often hurts), but it is transformative and life-changing. Carefronting our inner world means that when we are confronted with hard things in the outside world, we're more able to control our stress responses.

When we are stressed, the amygdala (the stress sensor in the brain) triggers cortisol to flood through the body. Cortisol stops us from thinking rationally about our actions and reactions.

Stress is a fight, flight or freeze response, and if we don't limit stress, we can end up operating in stress response too much of the time. This makes us sick and stuck. When we're stressed, muscles tighten and we experience raised blood pressure, indigestion, aches and pains, tunnel vision, reduced empathy, reduced intake of breath and a churning stomach. Over time, our sympathetic (fight or flight) nervous system becomes dominant, disallowing our parasympathetic (rest and digest) nervous system from doing its work in repairing and nurturing us to optimal health.

The dis-ease we feel is not only a progression to disease, but often means days off work and even job loss. Approximately 13.7 million working days are lost each year in the UK as a result of work-related illness at a cost of £28.3 billion per year – *National Institute for Health and Clinical Excellence, 2022.*

## DON'T IGNORE YOUR RED FLAGS

Your body is constantly giving you feedback and telling you what it needs. It's ever inviting you to notice your red flags (snapping at the kids, heartburn, dizziness, reduced quality of sleep). It's important to take the journey inward to explore those vital signals.

**Why?**

Your body wants to help you understand yourself. It wants to help you confront or reframe the things that are hurting you and keeping you stuck. Your body wants you to live well.

**How?**

Primarily, by being more honest with yourself, loving yourself and being kind to yourself in an authentic way.

## REFRAME THE PROBLEM

'The way we think about a problem is often more of a problem than the problem itself', Steve Backlund. Whilst it often feels like it, we are not tied to treadmills and can do something about our problems. Often, we don't because facing them is a thought worse than death.

We can change the way we think about our problems and invite different perspectives. We can also stop running and get off the treadmill altogether.

---

'The way we think about a problem is often more of a problem than the problem itself' - *Steve Backlund*

---

Take some time to identify your problem(s). What is your treadmill; Is it a person, a place or a thing making you feel stuck? What is the worst that could happen if you got off? What might happen if you stayed on?

_____
_____
_____
_____
_____
_____
_____
_____

## RESPOND DON'T REACT

The more we get to know ourselves, the better we respond to stimuli and circumstances, and when we do, our prefrontal cortex does its job properly regulating the body's stress response in healthy ways.

Our body is no longer constantly flooded with cortisol. We desire healthier outcomes, so our aim in step 4 is to begin to respond to ourselves (and others) rather than react on impulse anymore.

As we prepare to enter our inner world, remember why we are doing this, as it may feel uncomfortable:

We are going there to access our feelings, acknowledge our needs, process uncomfortable sensations and actively embrace the healing of our mind, body and soul. We do this by facing our discomfort.

- In this place, we find new and innovative tools to help locate and repair the heart wounds that make us act out.
- We are going there to have more honest conversations with ourselves.
- We enter to undergo the process of real transformation in life. No more 'fake it 'til we make it' attributes.
- We want to become more real and less robotic.
- We want to discover how to change our life for the better.
- We want to understand the importance of stopping trying to change other people, but instead spend time working on ourselves.

It's the place where we become unstuck from the challenging feelings that hold us back in life. It's the place where the light breaks through; the place where you check in with yourself.

## CHECK IN WITH YOURSELF REGULARLY THROUGHOUT THE DAY

How are you today? How is your head? How is your heart? How is your gut?

When your mind is struggling to make sense of something (huh?), your brain is signalling that something isn't right. When your heart hurts (ouch!), your body is telling you that something is off. And when you get that sick feeling in your stomach (eek!!), your gut is speaking volumes to you.

Step 4 is to listen to these signals and not ignore them.

The ways our head, heart and gut communicate with us are different for all of us. This is because some of us are feelers and others are logical thinkers; nevertheless, we all experience all 3 ways of receiving information.

## THE HEAD PROCESSES INFORMATION LIKE THIS:

'I'm trying to make sense of this and it feels like my brain is working hard. I'm overthinking. I'm intellectualising. I'm overtrying. I'm reasoning here. I'm rationalising'.

Notice what your brain is telling you today. Is it time you stopped ruminating over the same problem or going in circles? Is it time to stop trying to make sense of something non-sensical and take time to process something weighing heavy on your mind?

I needed to do this when my brain was telling me to stay in my stressful job—leaving was the logical thing to do. I was no longer in a position to work such long hours, and it was making me ill. I suffered from stress and fatigue, working 13-hour days plus weekends, but logic told me that the good wage was worth it. Meanwhile, my heart was telling me to establish healthier boundaries. What is your body trying to tell you today?

## THE STOMACH/GUT PROCESSES INFORMATION LIKE THIS:

'This doesn't feel right. I have a gut feeling about this. I'm afraid. I'm anxious about doing this. I need courage. I feel sick to my stomach about this'.

Notice what that gut feeling is trying to tell you today. With 100,000 neurons in your gut, this second brain of yours has about the same number of neurons as in your spinal cord. It communicates with your brain via the vagus nerve and exists to help you love yourself well.

## THE HEART PROCESSES INFORMATION LIKE THIS:

'I feel badly treated and it hurts. I'm loving too much. My heart feels enlarged. It feels overstretched and painful. My values are being ignored. I'm being invalidated. This relationship hurts'.

The heart is concerned with deep things – your core values.

Notice most of what your heart is telling you as life works when we let our good heart guide us. Within these 3 brain spaces, the heart is at the centre.

The heart tells us if our core values are being harmed, invalidated, or damaged in some way. Heartache tells us we really do care about something, or someone. Our heart also tells us if we need to repair a breakdown in a relationship or forgive someone who has hurt us.

When we are holding someone down for what they did, we prevent them from moving forwards, but at the same time, we're so busy pinning them down that we can't move either. We'll look more at forgiveness in Step 10.

### GIVE YOURSELF TIME

Notice how this isn't a process that you can do with the television on or your Instagram to hand as a comfort blanket. Your security blanket is the wisdom and freedom to do this process. Personally, I ask God to help guide and love on me as I visit my inner world. You may like to explore doing the same. Alternatively, go to your favourite safe place. Give yourself all the time you need.

## THE DEEP DIVE INTO YOUR INNER WORLD

Stay in this place and notice everything your body is telling you. Lay down your blame thrower for a moment and be brutally honest about what you're feeling, whether you played a part in your problems or issues and what that part was, or perhaps still is? Forgive yourself and anyone else you may need to. Take time to listen to your head brain, gut-brain and heart brain. What are they telling you and are they asking you to confront and deal with some hard things? What is the one thing you can do to redress and heal that? Do you need to move away from someone – or closer to others?

## RADIATORS AND DRAINS

Life is full of radiators and drains. Radiators are people and things that give us energy, life and warmth. Drains cause us to feel stressed, de-energised and drained. Perhaps your body is telling you there are too many drains in your life. Why is that?

Perhaps stress has accumulated in your life because you won't let go of what you need to or because ego, fear or pride is stopping you from doing what needs to be done or changed.

Perhaps you drain other people? If so, be honest with yourself. Why is that? And what can you do to become a radiator, not a drain?

_____
_____
_____
_____
_____
_____
_____
_____
_____

Each time you visit this process, you'll notice your body telling you a) what needs doing today and b) what is causing discomfort long term.

*Facing the truth and naming the emotion or issue you're struggling with is 95% of the way towards resolving the problem – Tony Beaumont*

Don't beat yourself up if you've ignored the things your body was trying to tell you. You can thank your inner wisdom, and God for his guidance.

Most of us have never been taught to be this honest with ourselves and to confront our dis-ease in this way. If the dive into your inner world was easy, you'd have done it already. But instead, life taught us to cover up, blame and shame others instead.

## GOOD NEWS

"Facing the truth, and recognising the emotion or issue you're struggling with is 95% of the way towards resolving the problem", Tony Beaumont.

## FEELING AND HEALING

If you are struggling to name your feelings, you might like to use a feeling wheel – there are plenty online. Feeling wheels help us name and identify our feelings more specifically.

Once you know how you feel, you may instantly know what to do about it, or perhaps it's something you'll need to think about for a few days. That's OK.

Always do this reflective exercise at your own pace and trust yourself. Your body is your temple, and it is wonderfully made in such a way as to help protect and care for you.

## SOCIAL BUFFERING

The more you practice Step 4 the more empowered you will feel to love and honour yourself and others better. Caring for others and protecting them from stress is called Social Buffering.

Social Buffering refers to our ability to love, help and support each other through stressful times. When we show kindness and foster love, friendship, and community spirit, we buffer or protect each other's amygdala (part of the brain) from triggering the full-scale stress response and 'fight or flight' stress reactions.

In practice, social buffering looks like; showing empathy, listening well or giving a hug. Once we understand this and make a conscious choice to give ourselves and others the time of day, we naturally begin to care for ourselves and others better.

The fruit of this process is happier people and healthier homes, workplaces and communities.

# STEP 5: Have Braver Conversations with Others
## Clear the elephants in the room so you don't keep tripping over their trunks!

*'Ignoring facts does not make them go away'*
*- Fran Tarkenton*

**PIPPA**

*Gran had always called her 'my best girl, my kind Pip'. Pippa missed Gran with her jokes and wise sayings. 'Kill them with kindness' she always said. Except Pippa was starting to feel like she was dying inside. Her husband had worked late for months and she felt isolated, having moved town for his job. She missed him. Pippa cooked nice meals, bought him gifts and did all the kind things she could conceive, but it was no use. Distance remained between them.*

*"You're never here John!" she blurted out.*

*"I've got a lot on at work Pip. Besides, you've got loads to get on with here before the baby arrives," retorted John.*

*Pippa felt dismayed. She had expected a very different response and had dreamed of John saying, "I'm sorry to hear that darling; it must be hard. How can I support you?". But John felt stressed and fed up. He wanted his wife to care!*

*"Why can't you just be nice instead of nagging me!?" said John exasperated. "Why can't you say 'I appreciate all the hours you work, but I miss you in the evenings, John' as that would be far nicer Pippa. Stop nagging me!".*

*It felt too scary for Pip to tell John this truth. She'd feel too exposed.*

*So, the status quo continued...*

# STEP 5: HAVE BRAVER CONVERSATIONS WITH OTHERS

I experienced chronic stress in my work, relationships and motherhood, and it made me ill. I went from a healthy, vibrant young woman to someone diagnosed with fibromyalgia, post-natal depression, endocrine dysfunction, neck and back pain, chronic eczema, chronic urticaria, bowel problems and more. It didn't happen overnight.

I had an unhealthy way of avoiding the conversations I needed to have because I wanted to avoid being let go or abandoned, both at home and at work. However, healthy people admit 'I am not in control of everyone and everything around me, but I have courage and self-control. I manage myself and my relationships well. I am prepared to have the brave conversations that I need to and I accept the outcomes of those'.

Sometimes difficult, painful or abusive *familiar* things can feel safer than *the unknown*. In my own life, I discovered that they are not. My healing didn't happen overnight, but once I began having the brave conversations I needed to and making more courageous decisions, I was released from pain and disease mentally, emotionally and physically.

## DIS-EASE CAUSES DISEASE

Non-communicable diseases are one of the top 10 threats to global health (World Health Organisation, 2019). As a society, we have become accustomed to feeling 'okay' or 'not too bad'. It's not good enough to put our health in the hands of overworked health professionals with a mandate for disease management, rather than prevention.

It was my own dramatic healing that led me into the field of positive psychology, wellness and coaching.

## THE SCIENCE OF HAPPINESS

Positive psychology shares many characteristics with Health and Wellness Coaching. Essentially, it's about bravely exploring our limiting beliefs and perceptions, and changing the shape of our thinking, habits, actions and relationships for the better.

The Bible says, "don't conform to the pattern of this world but be transformed by the renewing of your mind,". There are basic timeless habits and principles that, if followed, protect our mental and physical health. Speaking the truth is one of them.

## CLEAR THE ELEPHANTS IN THE ROOM

Once we understand what our brain, heart, and gut are telling us, we find that we need to have some courageous conversations with those around us to express how we feel and what we need from them. For some of us, this is an alien concept.

We may have been reluctant to have the necessary conversations with our partner, siblings, boss, friends, or co-workers, but in doing so, we can remove a sizeable chunk of our ongoing discomfort, anxiety, fatigue, stress, fear, and frustration.

*Our fear of having the conversation is worse than the conversation itself*

Usually, our fear of having the conversation is worse than the conversation itself.

Step 5 is to take responsibility for having hard conversations. If we don't, we inadvertently give away our basic human right to freedom of opinion and expression.

Human rights include the right to life and liberty, freedom from slavery and torture, freedom of opinion and expression, the right to work and education and many more. Everyone is entitled to these rights without discrimination (Human Rights, The United Nations).

If we feel bewildered, it's often because we have given away our will and sense of self.

It's time to take it back.

## THE PEOPLE AROUND US WILL ONLY KNOW HOW WE FEEL IF WE TELL THEM

When we are invalidated, disrespected or overburdened in life, the person or people doing it need to know the truth about how they are making us feel. The feeling may be in our head, heart or stomach.

We have the right to speak the truth lovingly and tell others what's going on for us, so they have the opportunity, at least, to care and do something about it. Be prepared that they may not respond positively to your invitation to care.

Let's be honest. We haven't told them yet because:

a) We were afraid of ourselves. We silenced ourselves, so we had no idea how we truly felt in our inner world.

or

b) We know how we feel but fear they won't care if we tell them – and then what will we do?

or

c) We believe we are being humble and kind by not having the conversation we need to. We may even use religiosity, or our faith in God, to rescue us as excuses not to confront those we need to.

Fear so often holds us back from speaking the truth and keeps us stuck. Healthy confrontation enables us to make good choices based on actual information rather than on our assumptions or fears. It's healthy to choose healthy confrontation.

## WE CONFRONT OUR DEEPEST FEARS TO *KNOW* THE TRUTH INSTEAD OF PRESUMING WE KNOW THE TRUTH

I can easily assume someone is too busy to listen to me, or I can find out if they are. I can assume they don't care about me. Or I can speak the truth and invite a response, then know for sure whether they care or not.

Knowledge is power. It gives us the information we need. And allows us to make wise choices. It prevents us from remaining frozen and stuck in indecision, fear, and uncertainty. It enables us to gather awareness and then take action accordingly.

Step 5 is to confront others in healthy ways. To do this well, we need to stop:

- Denying - 'It's OK I'm fine!'
- Minimising - 'It's not that bad, I'm on top of things'
- Blame throwing - 'It's not my fault, it's all their fault'
- Rationalising - 'Her behaviour is poor as she has a lot on'
- Intellectualising - 'I need limitless volumes of information about this'
- Exaggerating – 'I create drama but I'm unaware I do this'
- Catastrophising - 'It's just too great a problem to fix'
- Distracting - 'Don't look at the problem, just look on the bright side'
- Disconnecting - 'The silent treatment and withdrawal'
- Spiritualising - 'I'll do nothing and wait for God to do it for me'

Be honest with yourself. Which of these things are you doing in your life?

How are these affecting your wellbeing?

How are they affecting your relationships?

If you have the brave conversations you need to, what is the impact likely to be?

How are you preparing yourself for that?

This may mean updating your CV, asking a friend to support you, scheduling a meeting, chat or phone call, packing a bag or making notes on what you want to say to the person or people.

_____
_____
_____
_____
_____

_____

_____

_____

_____

_____

## NOTHING WILL CHANGE UNTIL YOU CHANGE THE WAY YOU DO THINGS

It's time for a positive change because nothing will change until you change the way you do things.

In my own life, I had been taught to minimise and ignore emotional pain and illness, to be loyal no matter what and to await divine rescue if it was ever needed. However, I discovered that God wanted me to be braver than that, and to have brave conversations, like Moses and Queen Esther did. Their bravery changed not just their circumstances but the course of history.

Rising up, speaking out and walking forward help us cross our own Red Sea. And we are not alone. We travel together.

So, I encourage you to approach others, inviting them to care or not care about you, and taking their response seriously. While ignorance isn't bliss, knowledge is indeed powerful. Although it can be frightening and may seem like a thought worse than death, ultimately, knowing the truth is empowering. Truth, which is the fruit of brave conversations, shows you the way forward.

# STEP 5: HAVE BRAVER CONVERSATIONS WITH OTHERS

# STEP 6: Listen Well – The Good Listener Learns More
## You have two ears and one mouth for a good reason

*'When people talk, listen completely. Most people never listen'*
*- Ernest Hemingway*

**IZZY**

*It had been a really great night. Izzy and Jeff were feeling closer than ever.*

*Before couple's counselling, conversations about money had been terrible but 4 months on they communicated with more empathy and care. Gosh, it used to be awful, Izzy cringed as she remembered.*

> *"Izzy, I suppose you've been out shopping again!" accused Jeff.*

> *"Not this again! Why do you always think I do nothing but shopping!? Yes, sometimes I like to choose for myself a new top if I need one, but I don't need one! I haven't been shopping Jeff!" said Izzy.*

> *"Well, tapping a credit card never made anyone happy Izabel," shouted Jeff.*

*Today, things were so different. They'd both learned to bravely talk, and listen.*

> *"I'm worried today about the cost of living," said Jeff.*

> *"I hear you. I understand. I feel like that too sometimes," replied Izzy.*

> *"Sorry you feel it too Iz; I feel bad I can't treat you more," added Jeff.*

> *"I love you, Jeff," said Izzy. "The times we spend together cycling, walking, laughing and cooking are always a treat. Hey, let's cook together on the weekend?" she suggested.*

# STEP 6: LISTEN WELL

**S**tep 6 is to take time to listen to others well and respond better

Healthy conversations reduce stress levels and help us practice relating to others in healthier ways. Being true to ourselves and 'keeping it real' means being open, honest, transparent and authentic, whilst creating a safe space for others to do the same.

Rather than adopting the stress responses of fight/flight/freeze, we need to learn to get better at talking and listening to one another.

**BRAVE CONVERSATIONS ARE ABOUT TALKING AND LISTENING WELL**

Do you consider yourself to be a good communicator and listener or do you sometimes feel disinterested, unable to concentrate or unwilling to listen to others?

If you're honest, do you dominate conversations and try to bulldoze people into doing things your way? Maybe people run a mile when they see you coming for a chat as they can't get a word in edgeways?

_____
_____
_____
_____
_____
_____
_____
_____
_____

Brave conversations involve giving respect and expecting respect in equal measure.

What does a productive brave and healthy conversation look like where both parties are actively engaging and listening to each other?

- A time and place that works for both parties
- Mutual respect
- No shouting/raised voices
- No belittling/name-calling
- Staying on topic
- Mirroring back to the speaker what you heard
- Mutual goal of resolution even if you still don't agree
- Not using the phrases 'you always' or 'you never.'

## NO ONE'S PERFECT

Human beings are not perfect, so we all have conversations that make us feel stressed and overwhelmed. Step 6 is to practice, practice and practice listening. The more you take time to hear others and notice how people experience you and your idiosyncrasies, the more you grow and become the best version of yourself.

Even after an interaction that leaves the blood pumping, heart racing and head aching, we should take the time to reflect and figure out how to achieve a better outcome next time.

In doing so, we learn a lot about ourselves and the unhealthy tools we use to communicate; not listening, butting in, shouting, going off-topic, exaggerating or seeking to complain rather than resolve.

Perhaps these are keeping you stuck and unable to resolve issues?

Be honest with yourself when a conversation goes wrong, and don't 'just forget about it' or beat yourself up about it.

When a conversation goes wrong, ask yourself:

- Was it a good time for both of us?
- Did I really listen or assume I knew their perspective?
- Am I too easily triggered?
- Does the person remind me of someone who hurt me in the past and am I projecting that onto them (their looks or mannerisms)?
- Have I had enough sleep or was I tired and irritable before we even started?
- Did I exaggerate?

- Did I catastrophise?
- Did I go off-topic or put words in their mouth?
- Was I respectful and did I just listen or listen well?
- Did I yell and shout out of fear or frustration?
- What is my dysfunctional dance?
- What is the part I play in unhelpful discussions?

A 'dysfunctional dance' includes all the unhelpful words and reactions in unhealthy conversations. So ask yourself, what can I do next time so that I can be respectful, and maintain my self-control and sense of wellbeing?

- I'll listen more
- I'll take some deep breaths
- I'll stand in a power pose rather than raising my voice to be assertive
- I'll leave if it starts getting heated
- I won't butt in
- I won't put up with belittling comments
- I won't try to intimidate or manipulate to hush them up
- I won't wind the other person up to illicit a 'reaction.'
- I'll stay on topic
- I won't raise my voice
- I'll reflect back what I heard

The more we take time to process the ways we listen, think, feel and act, the more we take ownership of our 'self' and our own issues.

When we listen and respond well to others, we improve our outcome next time.

You may think you don't have time to do all this processing, but the truth is, you don't have time not to. In just 5 or 10 minutes of reflection daily, you can learn a lot about yourself and improve your relationships.

This process increases emotional intelligence, reduces stress and makes us feel empowered, more confident and increasingly able to move out of our stuck places.

## PART 2 ACTIVATIONS

## PAY IT FORWARD - EMPOWER OTHERS

**Step 4:**

Help someone navigate a difficult decision by sharing your fresh understanding of the heart, mind and gut brains with them. Explain that their brain, heart or gut knows what to do. Encourage them to listen to their body and be kind to themselves.

**Step 5:**

Practice having a braver conversation with someone every day. Practice, practice, practice to create a healthier 'normal' and invite others to do the same.

**Step 6:**

Listen to someone today as they talk and share with you. Don't be tempted to make it about you and help them stay on topic, reflecting back on what you heard.

# PART 3
# STOP LIVING THE PICTURE IN YOUR HEAD

You've been brave in having the conversations
you needed to. So now it's time to erase the painful past
to create a happier, healthier future

# STEP 7: SET HEALTHIER BOUNDARIES

# STEP 7: Set Healthier Boundaries

Identify the real reasons you say "Yes" too much – and start saying "No" more

*'In order to thrive and be successful, you have to be able to set boundaries'*
- Oprah Winfrey

**ANDREA**

*It was a busy week for Andrea. She felt frantic and overwhelmed.*

> *"Can you lead the youth work Sunday? We really need you and you're so great at it so please say yes" asked Ben.*

> *"Okay, yes" said Andrea, before she could stop the words tumbling out.*

*Her head throbbed. She'd had a busy week project managing her house build, working overtime and rushing to and from the childminder, who was increasingly annoyed at her lateness. Andrea's toddler had no routine as the builders had been in for 12 months. If she did have a spare second, she cleaned.*

*Her family lived 100 miles away and clients seemed to demand more of her every day. Her eczema was worse than ever.*

> *"Give me a break!" she sighed.*

> *"Have a Kit Kat!" laughed the postman at the door.*

*Andrea managed a tired smile.*

# STEP 7: SET HEALTHIER BOUNDARIES

As children, we soon learn that 'No' is a powerful word. Parents and carers desire compliant children, so when toddlers learn the word no, things get interesting. "Eat your greens". "No!". "It's time to go to sleep". "No!" "Do your shoes up". "No!"

Kids are good at saying "No", but then something interesting happens. As adults, we suddenly find ourselves saying "Yes" too much. Why is that? Especially when, by saying "No" more, we say "Yes" to protecting the things we value - our time, minds, bodies, health and capacity?

Saying "No" is easier said than done, so to start doing it, we need to be honest with ourselves and understand the *real* reasons why we say "Yes" too much. Saying "No" stops us becoming overwhelmed, overloaded and stuck.

**WHY DO WE SAY "YES" TOO MUCH?**

The answer is in our unhealthy levels of fear or love:

**I'm doing too much because I'm driven by fear**

or

**I'm doing too much because I love you too much**

For me, I was driven by both love and fear. My life looked a bit like this......Yes of course, I can lead on Sunday. Organise your event? Yes! Meet an extra press deadline when I'm already behind. Yep! Host Christmas? Absolutely! Come to your hen weekend? I'm there! Cook every night? Okay! Live in a building site with a new-born and a toddler? No problem! Write your website this week? When shall I start? I can decorate your house, do your shopping, collect your children, have you and your family stay for the weekend...

Saying "Yes" to too many things makes us feel stressed, over stretched and exhausted. It's just not the way we were created to be.

The world was created with limits, seasons and timings. The tide comes in and it goes out. The sun comes up and it goes down. The summer begins, the summer ends. You are also created with limits. You live in a world with X number of hours in a day and the ability to get done all that you should be doing, but not everything else too. I used to live for an approval fix. I wanted to please others and make them happy, but it made me feel exhausted.

## AUDIT YOUR CAPACITY

We should each carry our own load so we have spare capacity to help others too. If we spend our life carrying other people's back packs daily, we will feel bogged down and de-energised. The breakthrough in Step 7 is not just in admitting we do this, but it's in being more honest and reflecting on why we do this.

Some of the reasons we say "Yes" too much are:

- I love too much (Women Who Love Too Much, Robin Norwood)
- I am a serial people pleaser
- I have been raised to put others first and give little regard to myself
- I'm living a picture in my head which is unrealistic
- I compare myself with others rather than stay on track in my own lane
- I have FOMO (fear of missing out)
- I'm afraid of isolation or loneliness so I keep extra busy
- I'm afraid I'll lose my friends if I say no
- I have too much pride to stop doing what I do
- I'm afraid I'll lose my status if I say no
- My circumstances dictate that I can do nothing else
- I believe I have to be a pillar for everyone around me
- I need to suppress my own needs to help others with theirs
- I'm afraid there will be consequences if I say no and I will be punished in some way
- I am co-dependent. I tell myself and others I am helping others but I have an anxious attachment style rather than a secure attachment style
- I am a serial rescuer and rescue those around me, even when my help is not required. It makes me feel better about myself
- I believe I am indispensable
- I need to perform in order to be loved

Our family saying was, 'I can do all things.....' so I had convinced myself, and others, that I was more competent a diver than I really was. My PADI dive training was rusty and just because I told myself I could do it, that counted for nothing.

I said 'Yes' when I meant 'No'.

I had forgotten my safety checks and even neglected to turn the air in my tank on, so putting my life in danger. Worse still, I was panicking on the deep-sea dive, used too much of the air in my tank by breathing too deeply and needed help from my buddy to remain calm.

We need to let those around us know what our limits are. We need to first be honest with ourselves about what our limits are too.

**DON'T LET FEAR AND PRIDE DRIVE YOU**

Let me ask you a question. Are you doing all you do out of *love* (being helpful, having spare capacity and enjoying it), or are you doing things out of *fear*?

Remember, acknowledging why we do the things that made us 'stuck' is the first stage of healing and 95% of the way towards a healthy change.

What were you trying to prove all those times you said yes when you meant no?

- I am a good person
- I am a hard worker
- I am not a loser
- I am enough
- I am worthy of your time
- I deserve your love
- I merit your validation
- I warrant your attention
- I am worthy
- I am irreplaceable
- My value is derived from helping others

**THE MOMENT OF TRUTH**

You have intrinsic value. You are enough.

In my 40's, my "Yes" became a healthy "No". My boundaries had been bulldozed past breaking point. My dive tank had run out of air. I couldn't volunteer for or be crowbarred or coerced into one more thing. I could renovate nor build one more house. And along with my loving "No', my energy levels began to increase and I stopped experiencing the most severe symptoms of chronic fatigue and fibromyalgia. I laid down the desire for approval and learned to love myself well.

**SEASONS OF LIFE**

The seasons of life change. We need to make sure we are living in season rather than living the picture in our head and from a season we are no longer in.

I have a dog now (a gorgeous lockdown puppy called Poppy), so I can no longer go to meetings in London without some planning. I'm responsible for my dog. I'm also responsible for my 3 children, who (when I had poor boundaries) used to be 'hand luggage' whilst I chaired PR meetings or was onsite at huge build projects. It seems laughable now.

You can be a successful businesswoman, an available friend, a capable hostess, a fantastic mother, a doting daughter, a loving leader, a special sister, an adaptable team player, a kind neighbour, a community-focused person, and a results-driven worker *with* healthy boundaries. Consider your responsibilities and determine if you are over-extending yourself in any area.

_____

_____

_____

_____

_____

_____

_____

_____

_____

I no longer use any of these roles to rescue others, escape heart pain, keep up appearances, or compete with friends or colleagues. Comparison with family members (especially with siblings) can be utterly debilitating and if that is you, I'd like you to be released from those chains.

By saying "No" to something good, we say "Yes" to something better.

Maybe, you need to say "Yes" to some alone time?

**FLEX APPEAL**

Our boundaries are never intended to be rigid walls - they are meant to flex – and they flex depending on the times and seasons in life, and our capacity at different stages.

Once you become unstuck in this area, beware, you will need to walk around your boundary lines regularly because old habits die hard.

When you change an unhealthy boundary, don't expect people to like it. Be prepared to face some opposition but take heart in the fact that your new, more natural rhythm of life will feel glorious!

# STEP 7: SET HEALTHIER BOUNDARIES

# STEP 8: Recognise and Step Away from Abuse
## Don't lose yourself to love someone else

*"If something feels off to you, you should take that seriously"*
- Serena Williams

**ARUNA**

Aruna's husband stood over her in the hallway and puffed out his chest. His temples pulsated and his face was reddening.

> *"You're nothing without me Aruna! No-one likes you. You're an irritant. My mum never liked you. My brother hates you. Who would want to hang out with a loser like you anyway! You poncy snob. And when I no longer need you to change nappies and clean up the kids c\*\*p I'll have fun with them without you tagging along like a millstone.  Don't go away with my mates? You're joking Aruna! You're not my f\*\*\*ing keeper. I'll do what I like!" Anish said menacingly.*

*Aruna had been raised to honour her husband, and her religious community told her she must stay with him. She was a homemaker with 3 children so had no money or income of her own. Her family would shun her if she dared even mention the word 'divorce'.*

> *"Domestic situations are private matters" her friends reminded her regularly.*

*Aruna felt the baby kick and fought back tears as she prayed for strength and endurance.*

# STEP 8: RECOGNISE AND STEP AWAY FROM ABUSE

On one level, negativity looks like that glass-half-empty person we all know who is constantly complaining and generally irritable. However, at its worst, it looks like systematic verbal, physical, mental, emotional or spiritual abuse.

Some people don't want to change and it's important to recognise this and protect ourselves from them. Allowing the negative and dysfunctional emotions, words and behaviours of others to leak over us is unhealthy. It's important not to deny or minimise the truth about toxicity and abuse but rather to safeguard yourself and others.

Faith is a significant topic here, too as, having grown up in the Church, I saw too many times women being told by a religious community, 'I'm praying for you sister' rather than the much-needed signposting being given along with safeguarding support. This practical help does not mean 'we don't believe in healing and reconciliation'. It means 'we will support you and the hope you have, while you are in a *safe* place'.

Sometimes it becomes clear that the perpetrator is unwilling to change, become accountable for their actions, attend counselling or stop the abuse. Remaining in the situation, living on a wing and a prayer for change, or crying out for years that the harm will stop is neither healthy nor okay.

You have a right to live without being systematically harmed, hurt or abused, no matter the source.

Receiving abuse or negativity is exhausting. It breaks the spirit, breeds fatigue and causes depression, low self-esteem, sickness, isolation, confusion and a host of other symptoms.

We may have no idea this is happening to us unless someone tells us or reports the perpetrator. Or, we may be fully aware of the dysfunction but believe we have no option but to stay - due to pride, fear, religious beliefs, illness or many other reasons.

Homemakers may feel they have nowhere to go because of financial reliance on their spouse. Employees may fear finding another job as their confidence has been so eroded. Spouses of religious leaders may feel judged or bound by their religious community.

However, to endure means to remain stuck. We may hope against hope for a miracle and that the person will change, but our mental and physical wellbeing suffers when we don't respond to red flags.

We may live in 'fight, flight, freeze' mode. When we do, physical symptoms can include bad skin, migraines, bowel issues, weight changes, endocrine dysfunction, chronic fatigue and disturbed sleep. We are likely not eating well either and using other substances like alcohol or smoking as a crutch, which further harm our physiology.

Meanwhile, our mental and emotional symptoms can include low self-esteem, depression, addiction, chronic fatigue, confusion, cognitive dissonance, detachment, isolation and even post-traumatic stress disorder (PTSD).

## BREAK THE CYCLE OF STUCK

The person, place or thing causing us dis-ease and disease makes us sick, but precisely because we feel so sick, we conclude we just don't have the energy, confidence or wellness to change anything. We struggle to change jobs, change friendships, stand up to abuse, raise our children, move house or even be alone. We feel we have been eroded. We may even protect the person eroding us.

But when the fear of staying in that place becomes greater than the fear of leaving, we will move. Please don't wait that long.

Step 8 is to acknowledge the harm being done to you, step away from it and empower yourself with knowledge and understanding about the behaviour or situation.

Gathering awareness is your key to getting unstuck. It's difficult and often unsafe to do this whilst still in the job, friendship, situation or relationship. Whilst you may be able to simply move on from a job, in marriage, for example, the issues and options are far more complex. But your physical, emotional and mental safety must be your priority whilst you gather awareness about what is happening and the impact it is having on you.

Programmes like "Freedomprogramme.co.uk" can be very helpful and there are charities across the country that run in-person programmes and support groups to help you process what is happening to you and provide the support you need. The police have dedicated domestic abuse support officers and lawyers generally give discounted help and advice at a first appointment.

*Own and honour your story however hard it is to acknowledge*

In the UK, 2020 saw the Domestic Abuse Bill introduced to Parliament, creating a statutory definition of domestic abuse, and in July 2021, UK Home Secretary Priti Patel published a strategy to increase support for victims and survivors, increase the number of perpetrators brought to justice, and reduce the prevalence of violence against women and girls (VAWG) in the long term. This was coupled with a £15 million funding boost to tackle VAWG in November 2022.

In Step 8, rather than keep pushing through, you can own and honour your story; however hard it is to acknowledge. Give yourself lots of time and space to do this and follow the light on your own path. Do not let anyone dissuade you from gathering the awareness you need.

The subject of abuse is far too large to cover in one chapter, so allow me to define some key areas and topics you might want to explore further as you reflect on them and empower yourself.

**Intimidation**

This doesn't have to be verbal but includes shouting, glaring, sulking and even firing questions at you but giving no opportunity to answer them. If you are in a relationship of this nature, 'Living with the Dominator' by Pat Craven is helpful.

# STEP 8: RECOGNISE AND STEP AWAY FROM ABUSE

## Verbal Abuse

This includes name calling, including when said 'as a joke' or in jest. 'Loser, moron, stupid, incompetent, silly little thing, idiot and you can't live without me' are all examples of verbal abuse.

## Emotional Abuse

This includes being belittled, ignored, isolated, manipulated, coerced, controlled or shut out from gatherings and social opportunities. In marriage/relationship, it often also presents as unfaithfulness, or using humour to instil loss of confidence and abandonment.

## Common Assault

Physical contact doesn't have to occur for assault to take place. If someone persecuting you causes you to fear violence, then that is enough in UK Law for it to be called common assault, for example, if a person raises a hand or throws an object and it misses.

## Gaslighting

A form of psychological abuse where a person or group of people causes someone to question their sanity, perception of reality or memories. The person it is happening to often feels confused, anxious and untrusting

## Jailing

Being isolated by a person who sulks when others visit. A refusal by another to help out so that you are free to do the things you want to do and to socialise. In a marriage/relationship, this often involves moving away geographically or removing your community or friends.

## Coercion and Control

This includes controlling finances and/or other aspects of life. Removing freedom and decision-making. Treating a person like a servant. Assigning the menial tasks to a person. Treating someone like a second-class citizen. This may be interspersed with grand or generous gestures to keep you hooked on a cycle.

### Sexual Abuse

Abusive behaviour by one person upon another. Sex without mutual consent. Using sex to control another. Refusing or demanding sex in a way that is demeaning or unwanted.

### Spiritual Abuse

A form of emotional and psychological abuse. Coercive and controlling behaviour in a religious context. Manipulation. Requirements for silence and secrecy. Coercion and or control through the use of texts and teachings. The abuser requires obedience and such an authority figure can suggest their actions or decisions are divine, so go unquestioned. They put you off getting the practical help and support you need.

### Narcissism

A mental condition where someone has an inflated sense of self, a deep need for admiration and attention, superiority, a distinct lack of empathy and troubled relationships. A perfectionist with a keen dislike of flaws.  A person with a great need for control. They will often be significant others, like a spouse, parent, parent or sibling.

### Antisocial Personality Disorder (ASPD)

This term includes sociopaths and psychopaths which are conditions defined by a consistent disregard for rules and social norms, repeated violation of others' rights, charming and charismatic on the surface but with a general difficulty in understanding or caring for other peoples' feelings or needs. Aggressive or impulsive behaviour. Little guilt for harm caused to others. Use of manipulation, deceit and control. People with ASPD may have a powerful gravitational pull on those around them.

### Empath

A person who is highly attuned to the feelings and emotions of those around them exhibits empathy. While empathy is the ability to understand the feelings of others, an empath takes on those feelings at a deep emotional level. By its nature, this can make you feel stuck or overwhelmed in life.

Empaths are accused of being too sensitive, feel overwhelmed in crowded spaces and spending life physically feeling the anger, stress, hatred, fear, shame, or excitement of people around them. By learning about being an empath, they can shield themselves from others' emotions and use this gift as a blessing rather than a curse.

Empaths are renowned for knowing things others don't and for showing the world how to love well. Their purpose in life is to promote harmony and support the healing of others. However, they may struggle to create healthy boundaries, which can lead to martyrdom, victimhood, co-dependency, and chronic self-sacrifice. If you think this might describe you, I recommend the book The Highly Sensitive Person by Elaine Aron, PhD.

Unfortunately, empaths tend to attract narcissists and narcissistic abuse.

**Co-dependency**

This is a dysfunctional relational dynamic where one person takes the role of the giver and the other is the taker. The giver sacrifices their own needs and wellbeing for the sake of the taker. This bond can occur between parent and child, between friends, and between family members as well as in romantic relationships.

This type of relationship is very one-sided and the giver begins to seek affirmation from the taker for his/her decisions and may even feel (or be told) they can't survive without the taker. The giver becomes stuck. However, creating emotional distance is necessary for help and healing to recognise the abuse and rediscover that healthy relationships are mutually beneficial, providing love and support to both parties.

**FREEDOM FROM OPPRESSION**

Ignorance is not bliss; knowledge is power. There is an abundance of charities, organisations, books, and online resources available to provide knowledge and assistance in all the areas listed above, as well as national programmes like The Phoenix Programme for domestic abuse and Restored Lives for healing from divorce. If you are in imminent danger or your life is at risk, don't hesitate to call the police.

Much of Step 8 involves unlearning the faulty and dysfunctional teaching, values, beliefs and ideas which caused us to stay in harmful, unhealthy or even life-threatening situations.

Particularly if you are an empath, you may feel it's your job and duty to shine light and bring peace to your place of work, to your bully boss or partner. When peace and care are not received nor reciprocated, don't stay stuck there forever. Take back your peace and self-respect. Shake yourself down and move on. Healthy decisions that protect your wellbeing and health are key to becoming unstuck.

If you are married or separated, this process might include reflecting on the purpose of marriage and questioning the true meaning of promises or vows you made '...'til death us do part'. The promise or vow does not mean staying until you are emotionally or physically dead. God's design for marriage is a supportive, healthy union that models how to love well – loving each other, children and society.

The vow alludes to facing and overcoming the hard things in life together. It does not allude to tolerating abuse. It is not an arrangement or a prison where one party suffers oppression.

In such cases the tragedy is not a divorce but the toxic relationship a person remains stuck in with the blessing and encouragement of those around them, and a lack of intervention in supporting the suffering party to get to safety while the issues are addressed.

The Church in the UK needs more reform in this area but is waking up and becoming better equipped to handle abuse more appropriately. Charities like Restored help train churches to recognise, prevent and respond to instances of domestic abuse. There is a global need to redress the religiosity and faulty teaching that causes people to remain stuck in abusive and dangerous situations.

## JUSTICE BRINGS EMOTIONAL AND PHYSICAL PEACE

Tolerating any injustice or tyranny can lead us to feel powerless, worthless, guilty or ashamed. This is because justice is like a fast-flowing stream of water that erodes the muddy banks of hopelessness to create new rivers of life. Align yourself with hope and justice, and you awake your parasympathetic nervous system (rest and digest) so the body can transition from its bewildered state of anger, pain, frustration and trauma to a state of inner peace and healing.

In my youth, I went through a period of regular hospital appointments for a chronic health condition, which led to me being let go from a job I loved. I had invested years of my life into the company, so on the day I left, I just wanted to crawl into bed and stay there. I felt sucker-punched. However, something else happened. Knowing that standing up for myself would also protect others gave me the moral motivation to challenge the situation and bring about a healthier outcome. The company in question settled out of court.

Having things made right not only healed my mind and body but also changed the accepted status quo for others too. So if you are facing very hard things today, remember that standing up for justice may change the course of history.

What is the one thing you can do today that represents a healthy "no" to whatever you have been tolerating? It may be big or small, but either way, it's significant. How will this decision help you? How will it help others too?

# STEP 9: Know the Difference Between your Core Values and Core Beliefs

Core values are not interchangeable with beliefs or preferences

*'Open your arms to change but don't let go of your values'*
- Dalai Lama

**CHRISTIANA**

*Christiana loved exercising. 'Movement is medicine' she always said, and fitness was one of her core values. It made her feel great and protected her mind, body and spirit. Walking cleared her head. Running kept her heart healthy. Swimming toned her muscles. When she exercised, she felt alive, so she prioritised it in her busy schedule.*

*Except she didn't.*

*Yes, Christiana believed in exercise and she certainly couldn't argue with the science behind it. But the truth was, she rarely found time to work out and prioritised her voluntary work at the Wildlife Trust. The session with her wellness coach was life changing.*

> *"Gosh yes, I do protect the things that are important to me! I protect and value wildlife but don't create time to exercise" she said.*

*Christiana realised that what she thought was a core value (fitness) was actually just a belief she aspired to live by.*

*Her growing awareness, about the distinction between values and beliefs, felt freeing. It shone light on the truths and lies she unknowingly lived by, and helped her become more wholehearted.*

**W**here we fit in life is determined largely by our core values.

Many of us use the terms 'beliefs' and 'values' interchangeably in life, thinking they are the same thing, but they are not. Understanding the difference between them is another step away from feeling stuck and towards freedom.

## WHAT ARE CORE VALUES?

Core values are deeply held beliefs that are unlikely to change. For example, I believe in God, I value justice, I value family time, I value harmony and unity, I value community, and I value lasting joy over momentary highs or pleasures that can cause pain.

Our core values make us who we are and influence what we do and where we invest our time and energy. They are our non-negotiables in life.

## WHAT ARE CORE BELIEFS?

Beliefs are ideas and concepts which can change as we learn and grow. For example, 'I believe driving is the best way to get around', but then one day, I may change this core belief and decide cycling is the best method of transport, as I come to understand the importance of health and fitness.

## WHO DO YOU THINK YOU ARE?

So often, we think we are living life according to our core values, but really we are living according to our beliefs or preferences. How do we know the difference?

We can quickly and easily know the difference because we protect the things and people that are very important to us.

I may *think* I value family time, but I may not, in reality, spend much time with my children, so it is not a core value but a belief I aspire to live by.

I may *think* my core value is healthy eating, but in reality, if I eat sugary snacks, this value is really a belief I aspire to live by rather than a core value.

Our actual core values are the values that we do live by. Examples may include; I am faithful to my spouse, I recycle to live sustainably, I volunteer to promote health and healing for others, I self-reflect daily to grow my emotional intelligence, and I value meaningful conversations.

When we live by and project our core values, we attract the life-giving friendships, careers and meaningful connections we desire. Whereas when we live by beliefs that dictate what we think we could or should be doing, we can end up living superficially and attract superficial connections.

## EXAMPLE

Dani Simpson: I value harmony, authenticity, healing, my faith in God, health and self-development, so I spend my time growing my body, mind and spirit, relating with leaders in these fields, and mentoring and coaching others. I also have a mentor with whom I check in regularly and to whom I am accountable.

I believe that I can improve my health by changing my thought life and diet, and by following a sugar balancing programme to eliminate glucose highs and crashes, and to stave off conditions like type 2 diabetes. My learning in this area is ever-growing and changes my lifestyle accordingly.

Write your own name and statement describing what your non-negotiable core values and beliefs are. Come back to and amend this statement at any time. As you gather awareness in life and your beliefs and preferences change accordingly, your core values remain the same.

_____

_____

_____

_____

_____

_____

_____

_____

_____

Step 9 is a wakeup call to many of us, and once we've defined our own core values, we can challenge those around us to do the same. In doing so, we straighten each other's crowns. We create families, friendships and workplaces of authentic people rather than wooden or robotic people who camouflage who they really are.

## CAMOUFLAGING

In my late teens, I noticed something profound.

If someone asked me a question, I would answer it differently based on which friend was asking, not what the question was. It was both draining and unnecessary. I was camouflaging many things and either bending the truth about my core values or dismissing my own thoughts and opinions to be more acceptable to them and theirs. Why?

I wanted to fit in. I wanted acceptance.

As a child, I'd been raised in a loving home and had all the ingredients to be physically healthy and academically strong. But like many children of our generation, we were told what to think and not *how* to think.

If our home is run as a tight ship, there is little room to explore our innermost thoughts and feelings and no safe place to unpack them. So as children, we turn to our friends, teen magazines and celebrity culture for guidance.

These influences and peers are powerful and if their high beliefs differ from our own, we can end up feeling isolated unless we join ranks with them and theirs. Standing our own ground confidently isn't necessarily something we've been taught to do, but it's something we need to do in life. We can always learn how to think for ourselves and develop resilience and a strong sense of self. We can start today.

## GOOD FRIENDS AGREE TO DISAGREE

We may have a belief that we need to agree with our peer group to be true friends. But good friends agree to disagree.

One of my closest friends and I disagree on climate change and religion, but we deeply love and respect each other and our differences.

91

## STEP 9: KNOW THE DIFFERENCE BETWEEN VALUES & BELEIFS

You are 'free to be'.

- How are you today?
- Who are you today?

While the answer to the first question will change from day to day, the answer to the second should not change. Sunday, I'm this person. Monday, I'm that person. Saturday night I'm someone else....?

In order to build authentic, meaningful relationships, we need to turn up consistently as our authentic selves, be present, own our story, know our own values, thoughts, needs and feelings, and communicate them clearly.

**WHO IS THE SAFEST PERSON YOU KNOW?**

The safest people we know are those who let us know exactly where they stand. We are aware of their likes and dislikes, what they agree and disagree with, where they will or won't go, and what they will or won't do. Their boundaries are clear, and we understand who they are and what they stand for.

On the other hand, we tend to feel unsafe around people who have soft boundaries and make statements such as "I don't mind, whatever you want." They may also change their minds, beliefs, or opinions when it suits them. As a result, we don't really know who they are, what they allow, where they're going, or what they're truly thinking.

The safest person you know should be *you*.

## PART 3 ACTIVATIONS

### PAY IT FORWARD - EMPOWER OTHERS

**Step 7:**

Free yourself from saying 'yes' too much. If they allow you to overstep their boundaries, they are likely allowing others to as well. Be honest with yourself and them, then encourage them to keep healthier boundaries.

**Step 8:**

Have a quiet word with anyone you sense may be experiencing toxicity or abuse and encourage them to get help and support. Knowing they are not alone can make all the difference.

**Step 9:**

Ask friends and family what their core values and core beliefs are. Do they know the difference? Which core values do you share?

# STEP 9: KNOW THE DIFFERENCE BETWEEN VALUES & BELEIFS

# PART 4
# THE POWER OF MEANINGFUL CONNECTION

You have now created space for healthy connections, meaningful friendships and loving relationships. These are scientifically proven to nourish your soul for optimal health and wellness. These steps are a hugely positive move away from life-less-ness and towards vitality.

# Step 10: PURSUE MEANINGFUL CONNECTION

# STEP 10: Pursue Meaningful Connection
## Practice vulnerability and authenticity

*"Vulnerability is the birthplace of love, belonging, joy, courage, empathy, and creativity. It is the source of hope empathy, accountability, and authenticity"*
- Dr Brené Brown

**PHIL**

*Every day, Phil made small talk with his colleagues. He often commented on the weather and asked his team mates, "Hey, how are you?", with little or no regard for their response.*

*"Good thanks, and you?" they replied.*

*They knew little about him. He felt disconnected and paralysed inside. Today his acid reflux was particularly bad.*

*"Come out for curry at lunchtime Phil?" Roger asked.*

*"Yes, sure," replied Phil. "It sounds great."*

*He was allergic to spicy food but it felt too late to say so as he'd been 3 times already. Phil was sick and tired of feeling sick and tired. He'd read somewhere that meaningful conversations are good for your health so he purposed to practice being more real with people.*

*"I'm meant to share my needs, true feelings and opinions, and not agree with people for the sake of it" he told his pug. Winnie growled. "I know Winnie, I'm not sure either," said Phil.*

*But as Phil began stepping out instead of hiding himself and correcting or judging others, he started experiencing meaningful moments. He enjoyed connections that led to deeper conversations. His stress levels were reduced. He felt less angry and developed more empathy too. Phil began enjoying life.*

# Step 10: PURSUE MEANINGFUL CONNECTION

**M**eaningful connection with others happens when we move towards vulnerability. Dr Brené Brown has spent years researching the power of vulnerability and she discovered that try as we might, we can't selectively numb emotions. When we numb painful emotions, we also numb our positive emotions. When we numb the meaningful and shut down vulnerability, we also shut down opportunity. Vulnerability is 'showing up well'.

## How Vulnerable are You?

Intimacy is fundamentally about vulnerability and having the courage to show up and be seen. New York-based coach and pastor Raymond Ramos explains that there are six levels of intimacy in our conversations.

1) Cliches (How are you? Fine, thanks)
2) Facts (It's so wet and rainy today)
3) Opinions (The team I support is the best)
4) Needs (I need your help with this, please)
5) Feelings (I feel disconnected from you today, let's talk?)
6) Beliefs (My non-negotiables are truth and transparency in life)

Our conversations determine the level of disconnection or connection we have with others. Therefore, it's helpful to view these levels as progressive steps towards meaningful connections and relationships. Level 1 represents the least meaningful interactions, while level 6 embodies the most meaningful ones.

True, meaningful conversations are only found on levels 4, 5, and 6. Unfortunately, many people spend their lives only engaging in levels 1 to 3, which can result in mere arrangements instead of genuine relationships.

## TYPES OF RELATIONSHIPS AND CONNECTIONS CREATED:

1) Disconnected Associations. For example, staff and customers.
2) Loose Affiliations. For example, parents in a playground.
3) Prescribed Connections. For example, staff in a team.
4) Connected Associations. For example, generic friendships.
5) Solid Bonds. For example, good friends and spouses.

6) Deep and Meaningful Relationships. For example, best friends and safe, loving spouses.

On levels 1-3, we show up but are not truly seen. When this happens, we feel disabled in our friendships, the workplace and relationships rather than fulfilled and fed by connection.

On levels 4-6, we choose to know and be known. We courageously show truth and courage, and develop clarity in life and fulfil our purpose.

Consider the important people in your life, for example, your friends, family, partner, boss and co-workers. Who would you say lives on levels 1-3 and who fosters meaningful connections on levels 4-6?

_____
_____
_____
_____
_____
_____
_____
_____
_____

Now ask yourself, how does that make you feel about them? How safe do you feel with them?

_____
_____
_____
_____
_____
_____
_____
_____

Some of us struggle to trust others due to trauma or life events, feeling that living on levels 4-6 involves dangerous vulnerability. However, despite our painful past, we can courageously become more comfortable by choosing to communicate our needs and feelings. This choice allows us to find new meaning in our lives.

By practicing the replacement of negative and unhelpful communication with healthier styles rooted in vulnerability, transparency, mutual care, and respect, we open ourselves up to a more fulfilling life. If we don't make this change, trapped feelings can begin to impact our health negatively.

## ANGER IS FEAR IN A MASK

The next time you are angry, ask yourself, 'What am I afraid of?' and use that as the talking point in your conversation rather than the fact you feel angry. For example:

I'm angry because I'm afraid. I'm afraid you'll never listen to me, never understand me and never resolve this!

I'm angry because I'm afraid. I'm afraid that you never eat your vegetables, and then how am I going to make sure you are healthy and have all the nutrients you need? I'm afraid you'll get ill or be under nourished. You need your micro nutrients.

## ACTIVATION

Below is a table covering 3 spheres of life (work, family and relationships) that commonly cause stress, frustration or discomfort.

In each column, a problem is identified, followed by the feeling created by the problem, a potential solution, and a meaningful outcome. You can use this process to reflect on issues or problems within your own spheres and then form a plan to pursue meaningful outcomes.

Keep in mind that completing this exercise requires vulnerability, but taking the risk is worth it in order to experience more meaningful outcomes and connections in your life.

## Step 10: PURSUE MEANINGFUL CONNECTION

1) Describe *how* you feel
2) Identify *what* or *who* the problem is
3) Reflect on *why* it is a problem for you
4) Decide *who* you need to confront (this is not always the person causing the discomfort)
5) Determine *what* needs saying and *how* you can more courageously solve this problem

As you go through this exercise, steer clear of using clichés and opinions or details of what somebody else says or thinks. Instead, describe your own needs and feelings, stay true to why it is causing you discomfort and find possible resolutions.

Remind yourself what your non-negotiables are (your core values) and choose joy, courage, empathy and creative solutions over and above your need to win. This is not about winning or losing. It's about finding the truth, and fostering meaning and connection.

| WORK ISSUE: | FAMILY ISSUE: | RELATIONSHIP ISSUE: |
|---|---|---|
| **I Feel Angry** | **I Feel Taken for Granted** | **I Feel Lonely** |
| 1)<br>My colleague is late 3 mornings in every 5. My boss seems oblivious to this. | My brother expects me to care for my niece and nephew every summer holiday. | My husband has a stressful job and I don't see him much because he's out with his colleagues or is at the gym most evenings. |
| 2)<br>My colleague needs reminding I have kids at home too and although I understand it's | I am in a new season in life and can no longer offer him this support. | I feel invalidated as I've communicated my desire to spend time with him in the evenings. |

difficult to be on time every day her lateness makes me feel disrespected and overburdened during the morning call outs.

3)

| | | |
|---|---|---|
| I will speak to my colleague about it. | I will speak to my siblings about it and speak to my niece and nephew to reassure them how much I love them. | I will speak to my husband again. |

4)

| | | |
|---|---|---|
| I will tell her she needs to be in on time. If she doesn't change I'll speak to our manager about it rather than continue to give her grace. | I will tell my brother that I have been happy to do this for years but that I am in a new season of life. I will be honest about feeling as if my help is expected and taken for granted. I will tell him I will help when I can. | Rather than say he 'always goes out' I'll emphasise my vulnerable truth - that I miss him and want to spend time with him. I will not deny or excuse his response but will accept it even if it's not what I want to hear. If he chooses not to spend time with me I will reassess our relationship. |

5)

| | | |
|---|---|---|
| My non-negotiable is that there is a change. | My non-negotiable is that he will need to make other arrangements for this summer. I can help on weekends. | My non-negotiable is that he invests in our relationship more than in his work colleagues. |

Healthy, meaningful connections don't assume that we are right and everyone else is wrong. To 'assume' makes an 'ass' out of 'u' and 'me'. Meaningful, vulnerable connections and outcomes bring our needs, beliefs, and feelings into the open. In doing so, we often discover that the other person has needs, feelings, or values that we were unaware of, and this newfound knowledge can change our perception of their behavior or our own discomfort.

We can best understand this concept by imagining meaningful connection as a rainbow. It is one rainbow, but we don't all see it the same way unless we stand and look at it together – our view may be obstructed by trees, buildings, or clouds.

As we move towards the other person, we see the rainbow from their viewpoint and perspective. We may find it is larger and more beautiful than the "part" we had seen from where we were standing.

**TRUTH SEEKERS**

As a human race, we need to become truth seekers. When we want to see 'the whole picture' and we want to value one another over 'winning', we build courageous, meaningful connections. We no longer jump to our own defence, anger, fear or judgements.

We can learn to talk in ways that seek mutually agreeable outcomes and get to know each other better. When we know and are known, we can connect.

Many of us have simply never been trained to do this in our families. Who shouted the loudest won! Or whoever sulked the longest got their way!

When we pursue meaningful, vulnerable connections, life is no longer about winning and losing but coming together to create connections and creative solutions.

Rather than argue, we co-labour, co-parent and co-exist well. Our sense of wellbeing increases and we don't spend time ruminating on propositional truths. We deal in actual truth. And we live in wellness.

Healthy communication is the outcome of good teamwork. When we choose to be a team, we enhance our skills and view others' perspectives, feelings, needs, views and opinions as important.

Respect breeds respect in our environment and life.

In this place, we also find we have fewer feelings of dis-ease or feeling 'stuck' regardless of whether we agree or disagree.

We choose to keep our love switched on towards others even if they don't agree with us. We also communicate our truth in love and if we don't want to participate, we tell others why not.

This communication style gives us fulfilment in our relationships over the long term and is more valuable than the counterfeit pleasure of making a point, punishing the other or 'winning' an argument.

Whilst winning might make us feel 'good' at that moment, it damages our relationships in the long term.

Do we really ever 'win' if it is at the expense of our relationship or losing our humanity or health to attain that win? Being at logger heads with others sends our stress levels and blood pressure soaring and is harmful to our health.

**KNOW WHEN TO STOP**

Conversations about which movie to watch are one thing, but discussing larger-than-life topics is an entirely different matter. We need to know when it's time to stop talking and take action.

Should we take our child out of school? Should we invest in an extension? Can your brother come and live with us for 6 months? Is it okay that the children witness what is now becoming abusive?

Sometimes, we can't endlessly discuss and reason about certain issues; instead, we need to make executive decisions in these circumstances. Drawing these lines and having these difficult conversations can be quite challenging. When discussions don't go well, we usually try again, but it's important to know when to stop. Continuing without a limit can cause damage to ourselves and/or others.

It's healthy to show honour and care towards the people in our lives, but we shouldn't let our commitment to others harm our physical, mental, emotional or spiritual health and wellbeing.

'Loving you and losing me' is self-abandonment and damages our self-esteem, energy levels and sense of wellbeing.

Whilst we should be able to flex (to be flexible), we need to ensure we are not always the ones flexing.

Realise that there is no right or wrong in many of our conflicts. In fact, most of our day-to-day struggles are not life-changing but purely a battle of the wills because we've seen that modelled to us by parents and care-givers. We can model something much healthier; a meaningful connection.

# STEP 11: Reframe Your Perspective of Rejection
### Rejection is simply a truth that someone isn't ready to receive you

*First publisher to turn down Harry also sent @RGalbraith [Rowling's pen name] his rudest rejection. They don't even want me in a beard!*
*- J.K.* Rowling

**HALA**

*Hala designed wedding invitations. Graphics and colours swirled in her head as she produced the beautiful styles happy couples might love. Sales were okay, but not great, and trade sales were low. She wondered if she should have given up her career quite so soon. It had all seemed so promising but six months in, she felt rejected and despondent.*

*Feeling the warm sun on her face she noticed an advert on the café wall. There was a short business course in her local area. The providers said they could help anyone succeed in business. 'Anyone' meant her. So, reasoning she had nothing to lose, she registered online.*

*"One last shot," she said to herself.*

*Hala never looked back. On the week-long course, she learned the vital importance of having a USP (unique selling point). By differentiating herself from competitors, she soon became the market leader of neon pink wedding invitations and rebranded her business 'In the Pink'.*

*She often imagines how life would be had she given up on her dream.*

# STEP 11: REFRAME YOUR PERSPECTIVE OF 'REJECTION'

J. K. Rowling offers hope to so many after receiving loads of rejections before her phenomenal success. Today she has millions of followers.

Rejection is one of the most powerful things that can control a person because we are created to live in love and acceptance. So how we view and respond to 'rejection' is crucial in enabling us to overcome it, heal from it and move on towards success. We can reframe rejection.

**REJECTION. HOW DOES THAT WORD MAKE YOU FEEL?**

Fundamentally rejection makes us feel 'not enough', but there's a much healthier way to perceive rejection which is actually beneficial to us!

**WHAT IS REJECTION REALLY?**

Rejection is a truth. It is the truth that someone couldn't receive you (or your vision or idea) because they didn't have the capacity to at that time.

Rejection doesn't define your value. It defines their lack of capacity at that moment. And capacity can be many things. It can be knowledge, faith or belief, wisdom, or even character.

Instead of telling yourself, "they rejected me," it's essential to speak the truth over yourself: "They didn't have the capacity for me. They lacked the knowledge needed for me. They didn't have faith in my idea. They didn't possess the wisdom required for my vision. They didn't have the character I need right now.

The same applies when we feel rejected at work, by friends or in an intimate relationship. Rejection is simply a truth that means that door didn't open to us, so we can wholeheartedly knock on the next door.

You may feel like rejection is negative, but would you really want your heart, idea, vision or value in the hands of someone who doesn't care about it?

We need to learn to trust ourselves, love ourselves and value ourselves. We can also stop seeking affirmation from others. This sets us free from the bondage and chains of rejection.

## STEP 11: REFRAME YOUR PERSPECTIVE OF 'REJECTION'

**FOCUS ON THE POSITIVES**

Isn't it interesting how as humans, we can have 10 people say positive things about us, but 1 person say something negative, so we focus on the 1 negative thing! Let's choose to change that. We can actively focus on positivity and joy. This isn't a passive thing. It's an active practice daily.

How can we practise?

- We can practice self-awareness and empathy
- We can start speaking up and stop being silent
- We can tell ourselves the truth - our voice matters
- We can choose to believe we're accepted not rejected.
- We can recognise that nothing will change until we change the way we do things
- We can recognise that our voice is hardest to use in situations where it needs to be used the most
- We can choose to keep knocking and keep trying rather than giving up

Step 11 says "Yes" to the invitation to live our best brave life, not our least hidden and fearful life.

If a door doesn't open, we can knock on the next door. We can ask for help when we need it and have no trouble helping others when they need it too.

These days I'm okay with receiving a "No" from someone, even if my feelings are hurt momentarily, I realise it doesn't wound or define me indefinitely. I learn from every experience.

**IT'S OKAY. I'M OKAY**

We need to tell ourselves the truth every day. 'It's okay. I'm okay. I'm acceptable. I create good relationships with healthy boundaries. I honour myself and others honour me too. I know when to flex. And I constantly grow. Rejection doesn't define me'.

Empathy helps us reframe rejection too. It takes us out of the realm of 'me' and into the realm of 'them'.

Perhaps they are very busy, too stressed, overburdened, overstretched or have no spare time for me right now. Perhaps they have a need I can't provide.

Empathy protects our mental health by fostering a better understanding of one another and enables us to be more present with each other.

It's how you show up those counts. When you know, you have shown up as your best, authentic, courageous, and vulnerable self, and they still rejected you it's much easier to accept that and keep moving.

## AGREE TO DISAGREE

Many of us believe that in order to protect friendships and relationships, we need to wholeheartedly agree with each other to avoid rejection. We think we need validation, affirmation, and acceptance of ourselves and our ideas, products, or viewpoints; otherwise, we feel 'less than'. However, we don't have to feel this way.

Instead, we can actively choose to keep our love on towards each other. Rather than concerning ourselves with judging, persuading, and changing others to come around to our ideas and desires, we can keep working on ourselves.

We then find that we start to attract what we expect and suffer less rejection as a consequence. We are more aligned with the right place, right time, right person or right people. We reflect what we desire, become what we respect, and mirror what we admire! It draws others to us.

Will you choose not to remain stuck in rejection? If so, this affirmation may be helpful:

*Every day I build a happier and healthier me, and I now understand that rejection is beneficial to me as I want people around me who are invested in me and believe in me and my character and ideas.*

*I move away from negativity and towards success. I don't stay in the place of negative thinking and 'not enough'. I choose to think in a way that is healthy and I have more empathy towards others.*

111

## STEP 11: REFRAME YOUR PERSPECTIVE OF 'REJECTION'

*I will not stop knocking on doors just because the doors I knocked on didn't open to me.*

# STEP 12: Evaluate, Prune and Grow your Friendships
## Choose who has a seat at your table

*"I have insecurities, of course, but I don't hang out with anyone who points them out to me."*
- Adele

**MEG**

*Meg adopted her usual spot in the jacuzzi. The girls were in high spirits and Debs congratulated Sky on her brave new choice of hair colour. As the twins exchanged notes on dermal fillers, waxing vs. threading became the hot topic of the day again.*

> *"No, I really think threading is way more painful!" winced Wendy.*

> *"More champagne, ladies?" the pool guy grinned.*

*Meg felt a bit lost. The good times rolled, but if she was honest, she wasn't sure how her friends had ever become her inner circle. They had little in common and seemed disinterested in her passions or ideas (she wasn't the least bit interested in theirs). Meg loved gardening and wanted the women to come hiking with her and Mike.*

> *"Let Mike the Hike go, and you stay here with us, Meggie," Helen had giggled.*

*Meg made her excuses and went off to read. Her friendships felt shallow, but at least she belonged.*

# STEP 12: EVALUATE, PRUNE AND GROW YOUR FRIENDSHIPS

How often have you found yourself in a friendship or as part of a group out of happenstance?

How many times do you find yourself with people or in situations where you question, "How did I end up here – with this person, in this place or doing this thing?"

Step 12 involves being honest about relationships that feel empty and unfulfilling, and questioning the reasons behind that. It's crucial to evaluate whether your closest friendships are purposeful or merely the result of happenstance. Consider if you've intentionally chosen life-giving connections with the people around you and if you have invested in deepening those relationships.

Sometimes relationships feel stale or shallow because we were not purposeful in choosing them in the first place, nor investing in them.

This can occur when we haven't been given permission to be ourselves in life, resulting in being surrounded by the "right people" that others have chosen for us. Alternatively, it can happen when we don't truly know who we are and attempt to fit in with people who don't really know us, nor do we know them. After all, how can they truly know us if we don't even know ourselves?

In healthy relationships, we should feel known, loved, and accepted. We choose our relationships. They don't merely choose us. When we share mutually healthy and fulfilling connections with others, we become unstuck.

**WHAT DOES A HEALTHY RELATIONSHIP LOOK LIKE?**

A healthy relationship is authentic and safe.

Emotionally healthy people share emotionally healthy relationships. They are their authentic self – no matter who they are with. They have nothing to prove. Their emotions, beliefs and decisions belong to them. They know, love, and accept others.

They innately understand their level of belonging in a relationship or group and have a high level of self-acceptance. This allows them to choose their friends, rub along with family and relate to co-workers well.

Rather than ending up in unfulfilling relationships and situations by accident as if life somehow 'happened to them', they feel empowered to choose their close connections and relationships.

They use their healthy relationships to practice healthy boundaries too.

People in healthy relationships feel confident.

**HOW ABOUT YOU?**

Are you being your authentic self in life? Are you camouflaging who you are to fit in with different groups? Do you emulate others to feel accepted? Do you copy your co-worker who has climbed the company ladder? Are you mirroring a sibling who seems to 'slot in better' with the dynamics and characters in your family?

To enjoy authentic connections with others, present your authentic self. Not everyone will like you and that's okay. We can't be all things to all people, nor are we perfect. Neither are they.

As we practice the 21 Steps, we learn that knowing 'me' helps me to know 'you' better.

As you evaluate and reflect on your important relationships, you will be asking questions like 'Are they mutually supportive, purposeful, and authentic? If not, why not?'

'What is the true motivation behind each of my important connections?' 'Am I friends with this person because I am using them for something or do I plan to use them in some way?' This is unhealthy.

**FRIENDSHIP IS GOOD FOR YOUR HEALTH**

Science proves that healthy relationships contribute to our good health. A study in the Journal Proceedings of the National Academy of Sciences showed that people with good friends enjoy better overall health.

A study published in the Journal of the American Psychosomatic Society, Psychosomatic Medicine, on loneliness and isolation revealed that people with affectionate friends perceive pain in a less intense way. In contrast, individuals who are isolated tend to experience pain in a more severe manner.

As well as decreasing feelings of loneliness, research from Duke University in the United States shows that people with strong relationships have better cardiovascular health.

UK researchers analysed 300,000 people and found a clear link between solitude and death. Other studies show that friendship can *halve* the risk of premature death, lower incidences of substance abuse and lower blood pressure.

## TRUST YOURSELF AND EACH OTHER

I deeply trust my closest friends and feel known, loved, and accepted by them. For years I forfeited that soul food because I was a perfectionist and the academic focus in my family valued performance over connection.

Performance-based love meant I performed and strived for those seated at my table. Thankfully those days are gone and it's farcical when I look back at how incredibly pressured I felt and how I tried to please the people I hadn't even chosen to be at my table.

## I'M FINE, THANKS

The 'me' I presented to the world was always 'fine thanks'. I thought my messy emotions were a burden that other people didn't need (they had enough of their own). I saw my emotions as tiresome, draining and time-consuming. I wanted to present to the world a businesswoman, mother and friend who had everything together and under control, who never felt self-conscious and wasn't ever preoccupied with what other people thought about her

In my youth, modeling had reinforced my insecurities when I didn't meet the stylist's or photographer's expectations. However, as a middle-aged woman, I finally said "Yes" to the heart surgery I wanted and needed. The skilled physicians were not consultants at various hospitals and clinics, but rather my close friends.

When I began being genuine about what was happening in my life, I was surprised by how my honesty allowed them to be more open about their

*What is the greater risk? Letting go of what people think, or letting go of how I feel, what I believe and who I am? Dr Brené Brown*

own inner worlds and experiences. Together, we embarked on a genuine journey. We had authentic conversations, and real friendships blossomed.

I was amazed how they didn't get tired of listening to or of loving me. And they pulled together to support me on Zoom, with coffees and with the time I needed and wanted. Was I really worth all that effort? Yes.

Are you worth it too? Absolutely!

Facing some of the real reasons we are stuck can feel embarrassing and difficult, but when we dare to face ourselves and our insecurities, we find true belonging in life. I know I did.

But that only happens when we present our true selves to the world.

There is no other way. There is no heart bypass. Is it messy? Yes. Will you sometimes wish you never started? Yes.

But richness in relationships is a gift that money just can't buy. It is optimal health for the mind, body and soul.

## THE BIG QUESTION

Professor, lecturer, and author Dr Brené Brown asks a great question of us all:

"What is the greater risk? Letting go of what people think, or letting go of how I feel, what I believe and who I am?"

Shame, pride and isolation are disarmed by honesty, trust, and connection. I'd like to leave that with you as you courageously reflect on Step 12. Remember, you *are* courageous. You are a warrior.

Thank you for reading this far and taking courageous steps to reframe your reality, challenge limiting thinking and bring positive change to your spheres of influence. You are a world changer and wellness in your inner world is available to you. You are whole, not broken.

## PART 4 ACTIVATIONS

### PAY IT FORWARD – EMPOWER OTHERS

**Step 10:**

Pursue meaningful connections every day with someone by inviting people to share their needs, feelings and beliefs. Encourage meaningful conversations on levels 4-6 (needs, feelings and beliefs).

**Step 11:**

Encourage a friend or colleague to reframe the rejection they experienced in a perceived loss or failure.

**Step 12:**

Give a friend permission to be real about their inner world and life by being more authentic and transparent about your own and inviting them into that space.

# PART 5
# STOP LIVING A LIE

With our healthy support network in place, we are now ready to embrace a deeper acceptance of ourselves and others. We truly understand that we are enough. So we are ready to pursue truth, resist payoffs and reject perfectionism. We are ready to fully embrace inner peace and balance.

# STEP 12: EVALUATE, PRUNE AND GROW YOUR FRIENDSHIPS

# STEP 13: Recognise and Resist Your Payoffs

Create cultures of honour; recognise counterfeit rewards and love yourself better

*'Everything I do is about women honouring themselves, treating themselves and taking care of themselves.'*
- Elle MacPherson

**SETH**

Seth's sister Libby was staying at his house again. Her brightly coloured suitcase and bags were strewn across the hallway and she'd already tidied the shoe rack. Seth grimaced quietly.

> *"Here, let me help with that and you carry on. I can get to school much quicker than you, anyway. It's true what they say, if you want something doing ask a busy person. I've got this, so don't you worry; I can sleep when I'm an old lady. Come on, give me the keys and let's get you sorted! Me and Daisy will have a lovely time together. You can get on with your work."*

*Libby's time was her own these days, and it increasingly meant that Seth's wasn't.*

> *"I won't take no for an answer," Libby insisted. "I love looking after Daisy, so come on or tell me where the keys are. I'll get them. I'm here to help you Seth," she persevered.*

*Seth wanted Dad/daughter time with Daisy himself. He'd been looking forward to school pick up. But Libby always wanted to make herself useful. She was behind in her studies and Seth wished she'd just get on with her own essays.*

# STEP 13: RECOGNISE AND RESIST YOUR PAYOFFS

Step 13 is to expose the payoffs in our lives; the counterfeit rewards that sap our energy and dishonour our very sense of self.

We tell ourselves they're a good thing, but they are unhealthy for us and those around us.

In simple terms, a payoff looks something like this:

1) 'I eat buttered croissants with jam for breakfast as it gives me a satisfying sugar hit (perceived good/payoff) even though I feel down about being overweight'. So the perceived payoff is actually unhealthy for me.

2) 'I help the Parents Association at school even because this alleviates my fear of missing out (FOMO) and makes me feel like I belong (perceived good/payoff). In all honesty, I can't spare the time and my business suffers'. So the perceived payoff is actually unhealthy for me.

A payoff feels good at the moment, but I suffer in other ways because of it.

I am deceived into believing the thing is good for me and that it makes me feel better, but overall, it makes me feel worse and is bad for me.

**CREATE CULTURES OF HONOUR**

Are the people in these two examples honouring themselves? No.

Are they honouring those around them? No.

They are unbalanced. We find balance when we move away from momentary perceived comforts and choose longer-term joyfulness.

Is the busy working mother honouring her time and the other parents? Is the lady eating buttery croissants loving herself well? What is the motivation behind their actions?

_____

_____

_____

_____

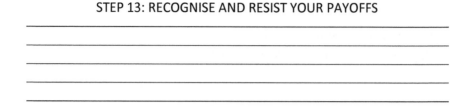

Both women are opting for temporary comfort or pleasure that harms in different ways, ultimately keeping them stuck. One remains at her current weight and experiences a sugar high and crash, while the other is trapped in her need for approval and belonging, regardless of the cost. The croissants and the Parents Association are not the actual issues; emotional pain is the problem. With some coaching, both women find healing, form new habits and so diminish the power of their payoffs.

## HONOUR IS A POWERFUL AND LIFE-CHANGING CONCEPT

When we honour ourselves, we are true to ourselves and honour others well in the process. Stephen Karpman studied human behaviour and came up with a model we call the 'Drama Triangle'. It's a great example of the dysfunctional ways we often operate as human beings and the unhealthy payoffs we buy into.

## THE DRAMA TRIANGLE

In the drama triangle, there are 3 roles – the rescuer, the persecutor, and the victim. In life, we all play these roles sometimes, and our roles change depending on circumstances. However, some of us get stuck playing certain roles.

We shouldn't be playing any of them, but when we do 'play out' these roles, the payoffs attached to each can seem quite agreeable. But they are not.

### The Rescuer

The rescuer doesn't honour themself or the person they are rescuing.

The sort of things a rescuer says (verbally or non-verbally) are:

'Let me help you, let me sort your problems, let me fix you, let me hunt for a victim to rescue'.

Rescuers can get very tired, but the payoff to them is 'I'm seen to be doing so much good' or 'by helping you, I can ignore my own problems and keep busy with yours instead' or 'when I rescue others, I feel empowered' or 'I'm in control of this'.

**The Victim**

The victim doesn't honour themself or others when they play the victim.

The kinds of things a victim says in life (verbally or non-verbally) are:

'Woe is me, my life is so bad' or 'you've got it so easy, and I've got it hard' or 'it's all so terrible'. They hunt for rescuers. They hunt for persecutors.

It's martyrdom.

Victims can also get very tired but the payoff to them is being surrounded by helpers, supporters, rescuers and cheery pom pom-type people. Victims are not taking responsibility for themselves and have lots of wallowing time (hippo time).

Whilst we all need to wallow sometimes, we can't stay there forever.

Gaining empathy and support is healthy (we all need some), but we can break agreement with the perception that *staying* a victim is useful to us. Partnering with a victim role leads to disempowerment, depression, fatigue and all manner of other health issues.

In my work, I see many people who are stuck here due to trauma. They haven't known how to process or reframe what happened to them, or forgive whoever hurt them. Forgiveness is a powerful medicine and we talk about that more in Step 20.

**The Persecutor**

Persecutors are extremely dishonouring of others

The kinds of things a persecutor says in life (verbally or non-verbally) relate to criticism and persecution.

"There's no hope for you". "Your potential is lacking". "The possibilities for you are slim to none". "Why do you do that?" "Why do you say that?" "Do you think that outfit suits you?"

Persecutors believe they are truly amazing and that others are unworthy, rubbish, less than or worthless.

The payoff to them is that by putting others down, they feel better about themselves.

Hurting people hurt people. So persecuting others is usually about feeling in control of or better than others.

In all of these cases, when we play these roles, we honour neither ourselves nor the people around us. It is unhealthy to play the role of rescuer, persecutor or victim.

**THE WINNER'S PYRAMID**

We can do something better instead. We can be honest with ourselves and visit our inner world to identify when we play these roles and why. Then we can flip the triangle on its head.

The Winner's Pyramid was introduced by Acey Choy in 1990 and showed how a Drama Triangle can be converted to something wholly more positive where win-win outcomes occur.

**'Rescuer' becomes 'Resourcer or Coach'**

**'Victim' becomes 'Vulnerable Creator'**

**'Persecutor' becomes 'Assertive'**

**The Resourcer**

In the Winner's Pyramid, the rescuer now becomes a resourcer. So instead of rescuing others, we show compassion by asking how we can help them. "What do you need from me? Do I have any resources that would help you? Do you have any resources that would help you?".

Language is powerful. These words let people know we are there for them and willing to help but that we won't give unsolicited help, smother them or take their responsibilities onto our own shoulders.

An example of this would be someone who falls and gets injured while out running. Rather than immediately offering aid with plasters, painkillers, water, or sympathy, we can ask questions to empower them with resources. Inquire, "Is there anything I can do to help? Who can I call for you? Do you have a phone, or would you like to use mine to call someone? Is my presence helpful, or would you prefer some space to be alone?"

### Vulnerable Creator

Likewise, the victim now becomes a vulnerable and creative problem solver. We all have times in life when we feel vulnerable and it's okay to admit, "I feel vulnerable right now", or "I feel vulnerable today".

We can let others know how we are feeling and let them know we'd like some help or support, or to be left alone. Rescuers can better help the vulnerable by becoming resourcers who are good listeners and team players.

### Assertive Challenger

Meanwhile, the Persecutor now addresses their unhealthy behaviour and realises that actually, people are okay. They don't need to put others down. It's okay for everyone to have great potential and possibilities in their life. In the Winner's Triangle, the Persecutor becomes the Assertive Challenger using their time and energy to help solve problems rather than blame others.

Choy's triangle enables us to operate as team players in healthy and supportive ways.

Name one or two of the roles you tend to play and describe the payoff associated with that role. What could you do instead?

_____

_____

_____

_____

_____

_____

_____

_____

_____

## DANI'S PAYOFF, 'KEEPING UP APPEARANCES'

I come from a family where we didn't confront or challenge inner dis-ease or disconnection, so as an adult, I used to maintain that status quo. Note how payoffs are often associated with family sayings, for example, 'don't air your dirty laundry in public', 'stiff upper lip', 'boots and braces'. Such sayings can be harmful if a person needs help or advice. 'A problem shared is a problem halved'.

I felt stuck on a treadmill that kept getting faster and I truly believed I couldn't get off.

I believed I had tried everything to combat dis-ease. Employ a cleaner? Streamline the business? Go on holiday? Manage the builders better? Employ a nanny? Drink more coffee? Come off rotas? Go to bed earlier? But, of course, nothing lightened the load or cleared the elephant in the room. It needed talking about. It needed airing. It needed sharing.

At the time, I unknowingly valued 2 things more than I valued my own mental or emotional health: 'keeping up appearances' and 'pleasing the religious community'. No one could know about my inner turmoil, and I was determined to avoid any situation where the truth might become apparent.

Unsurprisingly, I was diagnosed with endocrine dysfunction, stress, chronic eczema, and bowel issues, which led to numerous hospital visits for surgery and consultations. Why? I felt compelled to maintain appearances, stay busy, keep going, and uphold the status quo.

If I didn't, people would ask too many questions. I was afraid of the answers. And mostly afraid of the religious community who (as far as I knew) offered no practical option but 'long suffering' and 'endurance' for my situation(s).

But then I realised the truth.

I was responsible for being honest about my circumstances and seeking help. I was responsible for laying down the payoff, stepping away from 'keeping up appearances' and beginning the journey of healing.

By refusing to let that payoff go, my health had suffered significantly. In letting it go, I started to heal. Fibromyalgia ceased, my eczema cleared up, my irritable bowels regained normal function and I had inner peace. I didn't do it alone. I walked that path with God's help, and spent time meditating on healing scriptures, praying, noticing the beauty in creation, and spending time talking with friends, mentors, coaches and counsellors.

How we treat ourselves matters. You no longer need to set or maintain insanely high standards at any cost. You can connect with the deep part of you that knows how precious you are. You deserve the best care, utmost kindness and nourishment for your body, mind and soul.

**LET IT GO**

What payoff are you refusing to let go of?

How is this decision harming you?

_____

_____

_____

_____

_____

_____

_____

_____

## STEP 13: RECOGNISE AND RESIST YOUR PAYOFFS

You can't keep doing the same thing and expecting a different result. You'll only get the same result.

If what we are doing in life serves the people around us very well - colleagues, family, friends, leaders, and those we are in close relationships with, they are the last people who are going to tell us to stop. Even if what we are doing is to our detriment.

Today we can find and lay down our payoffs, and be honest with ourselves and others. We can live authentically. We have nothing to prove. We are enough. We can choose truth and lasting joy over momentary pleasure or perfect pictures. We can also even give ourselves permission to feel and to live a full life.

# STEP 14: Reject Perfectionism

Embrace your humanity; bravely face the root causes
of 'not enough.'

*"I've missed more than 9000 shots in my career. I've lost almost 300
games. 26 times I've been trusted to take the winning shot and missed.
I've failed over and over again in my life. And that is why I succeed."*
- Michael Jordan

**AMY**

*Amy had always dreamed of herself as an interior designer. She was
naturally talented and lent her creative flair to many friends' homes using
skills she'd learned in night school. But she didn't feel like the real deal.*

> *"We adore our new bedroom Amy," Elisha gushed. "The way you
> paired the cerise flocked wallpaper with the cream Silestone and
> natural wood was ingenious. I'd never have been that brave".*

> *"Thanks" said Amy. "It was nothing. I might charge next time…".*

*She wondered if she should have placed a larger ottoman at the base of
the bed. Amy watched Interior Design Masters and marvelled at how
Michelle Ogundehin layered colours and textures. She didn't feel yet able
to market her skills or gain big contracts. Her ideas weren't quite right.
Her swatches were a little off-key. Her mood boards could be better.
Clients might hate her designs.*

*So, she stayed in her day job while designers, less talented than herself,
secured big contracts for homes and hotels across London.*

> *"Maybe next time, I'm up to my eyes at the moment," Amy had
> responded to a golden opportunity from a developer, Octagon.*

*She was up to her eyes in the fear of failure. Every day, it cost her dearly.*

# STEP 14: REJECT PERFECTIONISM

Like Michael Jordan and Amy, I too have experienced failure, and each failure has helped me succeed. I've achieved success as a mother, writer, mentor, speaker, and healing minister, but in 2017, I ventured into the retail sector and failed.

I failed because I stubbornly refused to revise my flawed business strategy. I wouldn't admit that I'd made mistakes. I sold too many products in too many colors and sizes, making it difficult to keep track of my stock. As a busy mother of three, who was also building a house, I didn't have the time to devote to growing such a business. Moreover, my pride got in the way. I wanted others to see me as successful, not as someone struggling in the retail world. Consequently, I persisted for far too long.

Only when I stepped away from this perfectionism, did I observe two very helpful things happen:

1) I saw the business for what it was – a drain on me, my time and my resources.
2) I realised it's better to sell one product on a global scale, than sell many products locally.

Honesty with self (accepting this isn't working for me) helps us simplify our thinking, crystallise our vision, spot the lies we're believing and make positive changes. Failure teaches us to win.

When we are braver and more honest with ourselves, we embrace what we formerly perceived as 'failure' and recognise that each failure shows us the way to win.

## HOW DO YOU KNOW IF YOU MAY BE A PERFECTIONIST?

- You struggle to perform tasks unless done perfectly
- You view the end (the destination) as the most important part of the undertaking
- You have less focus on the process of learning, growing or doing your best. There is more focus on the 'perfect' result
- Procrastination is an issue as you don't want to start a task unless you know you can do it perfectly.

- You take excessive time to complete tasks that others complete in good time

## PERFECTIONISM

Many of us are perfectionists. We are stuck in striving, maximum effort, desire for flawlessness and performance-based love. But this steals our life, health, self-esteem, peace and wellbeing. It also stops us 'trying' new things in case we fail.

When we are perfectionists, shame is our biggest enemy and we live by the highest standards possible with rigid expectations of others and ourselves, all the while chained to our specific ideas about how things should be done, organised, or driven. "Perfectionism is not the same thing as striving to be your best. Perfection is not about healthy achievement and growth" Dr Brené Brown, Research Professor.

Perhaps in the past (or in the present), we have received punishment for failure. Perhaps we've been stonewalled or berated, lost something or someone we love, or even received physical punishment for not succeeding. We stepped away from such abuse in Step 8 and so now we can learn how to fail well.

Dr Brown explains that perfectionism is used as a shield against pain, blame, judgement or shame.

---

"Perfectionism is not the same thing as striving to be your best. Perfection is not about healthy achievement and growth" Dr Brené Brown

---

Whilst perfectionists tend to be reliable, they are commonly overly anxious and critical when expectations are not met whether at work, at home or in romantic relationships.

I was a perfectionist and still struggle with perfectionism sometimes because old habits die hard. It's a trait that gives a powerful drive to succeed and increases the chances of being a high achiever in life. But it also comes with self-defeating thoughts and limiting rigid behaviours that can make it harder to achieve goals. Simple tasks can take a long time to complete.

## PERFECTIONISM IS PAINFUL

Whilst I was a straight-A student and went to a top university, my cohort seemed to soar through each week while I lost hours of time making my assignments 'perfect'. It was a painful process.

I'm trying not to repeat that process 25 years on as I write this book; I'm actually wondering what I've left out that would have been more helpful to you. Yes, I'm still on this journey!

Perfectionists tend to have a lot of self-criticisms and feel inadequate. I often used the term 'healthy perfectionism' to justify my perfectionist traits. But perfectionism is not healthy. Nor is the belief that perfection is even achievable.

The journey of life is the destination. So, you are already there. Me too.

The result then matters less. Rather, how we give and receive love matters. How well we have grown our emotional intelligence matters. How we honour ourselves and those around us matters. How compassionate we are matters. How mindful and present we are matters. It all matters.

None of these things are - nor ever can be - perfect.

## BREAK THE PRISON WALLS OF PERFECTIONISM

Step 14 is to lay down perfectionism and embrace life. How? We can courageously face the root issues of 'not enough' or 'performance-based love' in our life.

Life is enriched when we are proud of our progress, satisfied by our learning, happy about our hard work and okay with finding beauty in brokenness.

## STEP 14: REJECT PERFECTIONISM

How debilitating it is to spend an hour writing a quick email! To believe you've failed if you don't get 100% in a test. To struggle to champion others easily. To compare yourself to others. To skip things you wouldn't have a go at in case perfection isn't achieved or to fear being shown up. How sad to focus on results only, losing the joy of the journey itself.

If you can conquer Step 14, you are saved from a life of excessive stress and burnout. You are less likely to develop harmful habits to cope with stress, and you will start feeling energised, not overwhelmed in life.

The goals you set for yourself can then become exciting rather than intimidating or frightening.

Hopelessness becomes hopefulness and the risk factors of self-criticism, self-harm and self-sabotage are uprooted by the freedom to fail. And fail; you must to overcome this.

Instead of telling yourself, 'I've got to do all this perfectly,' you can say, 'I get to do all this', and enjoy the journey.

# STEP 15: Stop Being a False Peacekeeper
## Move from conflict avoidance to genuine understanding and peaceful solutions

*"Imagine all the people living life in peace. You may say that I'm a dreamer, but I'm not the only one. I hope someday you'll join us and the world will be as one."*
*- John Lennon*

**BOB**

Jen felt utterly bewildered with all the pretence in the room. It felt so surreal and exasperating.

> *"Hey come on, don't rock the boat Jen it's really not worth it, is it sweetheart? I think we can all safely say there's no big problem here. Let's just have a nice holiday together," Bob smiled.*

> *"How can we have a nice holiday!?" exclaimed Jen. "So, we all just pretend what you've done never happened and hope it won't continue to happen, right under our noses!? Hello? Have none of you got anything to say? Don't you even care?".*

*No-one said a word. A couple of the lads shifted uneasily and everyone avoided making eye contact with Jen. Jen was in disbelief. The room seemed to be swimming.*

> *"Come on now Jen I'm sure like me and everyone here, you just want us all to have a nice time together. Let's just forget this was ever mentioned. We'll be all the better for it. The taxis will be outside in 3 minutes. Great! It looks like we're all agreed then" said Bob*

# STEP 15: STOP BEING A FALSE PEACE KEEPER

.

E veryone loves a 'peacekeeper,' but there's a world of difference between a genuine article and a counterfeit. Counterfeit peace is merely conflict avoidance. Many of us find ourselves stuck in life because we are counterfeit peacekeepers.

Peace is not the absence of conflict; it's the ability to handle it in peaceful ways.

When we act as false peacekeepers, whether knowingly or unknowingly, we may appear genuine but often contribute to a dysfunctional and counterproductive peace. Although we assert a great emphasis on peace, our actual objective is to achieve 'an absence of conflict at any cost'.

In pursuit of this goal, we resort to pretense, concealment, and manipulation. We brush issues under the rug and embellish situations to appease and pacify those around us.

We are stuck because we are deceiving ourselves and others.

You are a false peacekeeper if you:

a) Do things to keep others happy. You are a serial people pleaser and keeping people happy is more important to you than challenging your dysfunctional relationships and limiting beliefs.

b) You avoid doing what is right to avoid tension. You maintain mediocrity by failing to make tough decisions people may not like.

c) You hope problems will go away or others will make the tough decisions for you.

d) You avoid confrontation at all costs.

e) You condemn others rather than confront issues.

f) You lack the humility required to create an environment for restoration. You won't engage in conversation humbly, owning your own part in the problem.

g) You reflect the temperature and temperament in the room even if you know it should and could be different.

h) You value the status quo and favour unity over courageously discussing sensitive subjects.

i) You fear losing someone more than you fear never growing in this area.

# STEP 15: STOP BEING A FALSE PEACE KEEPER

False peacekeeping oversteps the boundaries of healthy, emotionally intelligent living, venturing into the realms of fearful living. It is the opposite of all we admire about individuals who have stood tall as genuine peace makers. People like Mother Theresa, Martin Luther King Jr, Nelson Mandela and those you know who create atmospheres for discussion, healing and restoration. Their peace-making efforts require conviction, diligence, perseverance, humility and grace.

## Are you Facilitating a Dynamic of False Peacekeeping Fuelled by Fear?

Living within this dysfunctional dynamic cultivates a fear of confrontation and rejection. It's essential to adapt and compromise at times, but the real danger surfaces when we yield excessively and too often. This also applies when we coerce others into adopting 'peaceful solutions' with which they do not align, or when we permit individuals in our lives to don the 'peacekeeper' mask as a facade. We may convince ourselves that we are preserving their honor or reputation.

However, enduring false peacekeeping often breeds layers of underlying resentment or pain. It paints a picture of individuals reluctantly 'dancing' with one another while yearning to exit the scene. It is neither respectful, loving, nor kind.

This is very different to being a genuine peacemaker who keeps the peace, arbitrates, mediates and reconciles adversaries in healthy, genuine and successful ways.

Step 15 is to bravely 'rock the boat'.

## PROPOSITIONAL PEACE

Being a false peacekeeper can be hugely enticing but it has a damaging payoff; propositional peace.

We tell ourselves and others that we have generated peace, when really, we have failed to confront the issues at all!

Many of us grew up in families where healthy conflict was avoided, or we have experienced trauma in life where confronting issues resulted in aggression or abuse towards us. Maybe we had alcoholic or poorly parents who taught us how to walk on eggshells at home and do all in our power to keep things peaceful and calm at any cost.

Are you a false peacekeeper? What can you do differently to change that?

_____
_____
_____
_____
_____
_____
_____
_____
_____

## WE ARE NO LONGER CHILDREN

We no longer need to walk on eggshells. We can quit both 'being' false peacekeepers and 'allowing' false peacekeeping. This character trait causes dis-ease in our inner and outer worlds.

We are fully empowered to 'pursue peace' and it is achieved not by force but by understanding. In that place, we find that our life becomes one in which anxiety and worry reduce, we have fewer headaches and we no longer feel so stressed or afraid.

We feel whole.

**PART 5 ACTIVATIONS**

**PAY IT FORWARD - EMPOWER OTHERS**

**Step 13:**

Identify every payoff. Honour those around you by being more honest with them about the real motives behind your actions.  Encourage them to do the same.

**Step 14:**

Embrace humanity by not requiring perfectionism from those around you. Actively let them know their efforts are 'good enough' and praise what they are doing well.

**Step 15:**

Pursue genuine and healing peace with someone by attempting to resolve a conflict that previously seemed impossible to heal

# PART 6
# LIVE – REALLY LIVE

We are now happier and healthier. We are ready to grow our emotional intelligence, gather deeper awareness through journalling, let go of fear and find a job we love

# STEP 15: STOP BEING A FALSE PEACE KEEPER

# STEP 16: Grow Your Emotional Intelligence (EQ)

Whilst we are born with our IQ, we can always grow our EQ

*"Always be a first-rate version of yourself, instead of a second-rate version of someone else"*
- Judy Garland

**MATTIA**

Mattia was unrepentant.

> *"Ah I was born this way, it's my fiery Mediterranean genes Alice" said Mattia as his PA tried to explain his clients' issue. "My father was exactly the same, and his father, and his father too. I'm impulsive, that's just me. I say exactly what I think, when I think it. I can't change that. If he's upset, he just needs to deal with it. How do you say....a leopard can never change his spots".*

*Alice sighed and shuffled her papers. She saw the sales team drive out of the carpark and heard the roar of engines down the High Street. The attitude of her boss increasingly riled her.*

> *"I cannot go around adapting this and changing that to make allowances for the way he wants to work with me. It is my way or the highway" Kenzo span round on his chair in the vast new office. "You will see, they all need to up the game Alice. No if's and no but's".*

*The car park emptied and the office was now still. Petit Panu the sandwich guy had clocked that few staff were around and so didn't come in. Alice had really fancied a tuna salad.*

> *"Where were we?  Okay yes, I need a flight for Monday," continued Mattia. "British Airways is fine".*

# STEP 16: GROW YOUR EMOTIONAL INTELLIGENCE.

E motional intelligence (EQ) is, "The capacity to be aware of, control and express one's emotions, and to handle interpersonal relationships judiciously and empathetically. It is the key to both personal and professional success" (Oxford Languages)

By Step 16, you will have reached a stage where hiding, shaming and blaming others for the hard things we couldn't face is no longer an option. We have grown. Every day, whether we're 19 or 90, we can practise living more intelligently.

## LOW EMOTIONAL INTELLIGENCE

Low EQ looks like someone who is argumentative, doesn't listen, blames others and has frequent unrestrained emotional outbursts.

If this sounds like you it's okay to be honest with yourself. We are here to become unstuck and embrace a happier healthier 'self' so you're on the right track if you said 'yes' to any of these low EQ indicators.

## HEALTHY EMOTIONAL INTELLIGENCE

When we consider EQ we focus on growing in the four main areas:

1) Self-awareness
2) Self-management
3) Social awareness
4) Relationship management

Daniel Goleman is a leader in this field and identified the following behaviours in people with emotional intelligence.

They: -

- Recognise and understand their own mood, emotions and motivations as well as their effect on others
- Control and redirect disruptive impulse think before acting
- Work for reasons beyond money or status
- Pursue goals with energy and persistence
- Understand the emotions of others
- Manage relationships well
- Build good rapport with others

# STEP 16: GROW YOUR EMOTIONAL INTELLIGENCE

## HOW IS YOUR EMOTIONAL INTELLIGENCE?

As we consider these four areas, reflect on where your strengths and weaknesses lie, and identify areas you'd like to grow in:

1) Self-awareness

- Emotional self-awareness (where you can identify and understand your emotions as well as recognise their impact on your relationships).
- Accurate self-assessment (where you can be realistic about your strengths and weaknesses).
- Self-confidence (where you have a positive sense of self-worth).

2) Self-management

- Self-control (keeping disruptive emotions under control)
- Transparency (living with honestly and integrity, and managing yourself well).
- Adaptability (the ability to adapt to changing situations and overcome obstacles).
- Achievement (the drive to meet your internal standards of excellence)
- Initiative (the readiness to seize opportunities).

3) Social awareness

- The social skill that arguable benefits our relationships most in this area is empathy; do we empathise with others? Empathy is very different from sympathy. Empathy understands the feelings of others, whereas sympathy conveys pity.

4) Relationship management

- This is our ability to influence others (listening well and sending clear and convincing messages), manage conflict (resolve disagreements and develop resolutions), build and maintain good relationships with others, and cooperate.

Which area do you feel you want to grow in and why?

_____

_____

_____

_____

_____

_____

_____

_____

_____

In any of the areas where we score low, we can grow thanks to honest reflection, a willingness to change and a desire to move forwards.

**TRANSFORM YOUR MIND**

Since the early 1980's, neuroscientist Dr Caroline Leaf has researched the connection between the mind and the brain. She was one of the first in her field to study neuroplasticity (how the brain can actually change with directed input) and the research is exciting.

Our thoughts, feelings and behaviours can be reconceptualised and changed. Our brains can quite literally shape up emotionally. What does this mean for us?

*"We are not victims of our biology. We are co-creators of our destiny......"*

*"We have been designed to create thoughts, and from these we live out our lives."*

*"You cannot sit back and wait to be happy and healthy, and have a great thought life; you have to make the choice to make this happen."*

*"You can be overwhelmed by every small setback in life, or you can be energised by the possibilities they bring."*

# STEP 16: GROW YOUR EMOTIONAL INTELLIGENCE

*"Our brains are wired for love"*

*Dr Caroline Leaf*

These statements challenged my thinking. Science proves that we can learn the emotional and relational skills that we are lacking at any age.

Dr Leaf explains, "...thoughts are basically electrical impulses, chemicals and neurons. They look like a tree with branches. As we change our thinking, some branches go away, new one's form, the strength of the connections change, and the memories network with other thoughts".

This means that by changing our thinking, we can reframe our feelings, and grow our emotional intelligence and learned responses.

## UNLEARN 'REACTIONS' AND LEARN 'RESPONSES'

Every day we face any number of toxic experiences or interactions; an email, a text message from a friend, a tough conversation or meeting, and so on. "We need to learn how to deal with such situations, not run from them," explains Dr Leaf.

Our true power lies in observing things with logic and restraint, not reacting to them with neither. Self-control, self-management and self-restraint are our superpowers.

When we can step back and observe or notice a situation, we feel more able to deal with it, rather than feeling overwhelmed by it.

Life is not perfect and intrusive thoughts and toxic experiences pervade each one of us with negative messages such as 'no one likes you', 'you'll never change', 'you might as well give up now', 'you didn't do very well' or 'who'd want to be your friend?' but we can choose to literally snap those branches off our thought trees.

## TOXIC THOUGHTS ATTRACT MORE TOXIC THOUGHTS

According to Dr Leaf "If you continually choose to give people power over you by continually ruminating over what they said or did, you will continue to suffer, damaging your brain and mental health in the process".

Suppose we have developed unhealthy patterns of low EQ, reacting to our environment and the people around us rather than responding well. In that case, we can easily get stuck in toxic reactions and mismanagement of our emotions.

Rather we can learn to develop self-regulation. The truth is we are not under anyone's control unless we allow it. We can't be offended unless we choose to take offence. And we have countless opportunities every day to respond well to others and practise growing our EQ in all of the 4 main areas.

Revisit your list of the areas you'd like to grow in and reflect on *how* you will practically do that this week. Where is your biggest EQ struggle? What can you do differently?

_____

_____

_____

_____

_____

_____

_____

_____

_____

# STEP 16: GROW YOUR EMOTIONAL INTELLIGENCE

# STEP 17: Find Joy and Value at Work – or Find a New Job!

Take yourself seriously – you're done with dysfunctional dances

*"The only way to do great work is to love what you do. If you haven't found it yet- keep looking. Don't settle"*
- Steve Jobs

**HARVEY**

Dave just had to know why Harvey remained so upbeat.

"How is it you're able to stay so positive in this place?" asked Dave. He'd worked at the MILO Hotel for 11 months and guests seemed ever more demanding.

*Harvey understood the difference between happiness and joy at work.*

*"Even happy staff have bad weeks and wonder 'Why do I not feel joyful and content?'" Harvey explained. "Happiness is a completely different state of mind to being joyful"*

*"You see, happiness can't be used interchangeably with joy Dave. Happiness is momentary. It's derived from pleasure or a fleeting moment, but joy is a mindset you carry with you" he smiled.*

*"But how do you find joy at work?" Dave asked.*

*"I'll tell you how Dave. Don't sweat the small stuff. Confront the big stuff. Do what you love and make the best of what you don't. Most importantly though, never confuse happiness with joy," said Harvey. "Find the joy".*

*"A job is what you make it. Joy and contentment are yours for keepers. No one can take them away. If you have the right mindset and you still can't find the joy at work, find a different job," Harvey beamed.*

**W**ork environments are intriguing places. So many relational dances, power plays and games go on there. But whatever the dysfunctional dance at our place of work, there is so much we can do to change the dysfunctional steps. We can also leave the dance floor!

Working hard for something we don't care about is called stress. Whereas working hard towards something we do care about is called passion.

Even the most challenging or mundane work environments can be made happier, healthier, and more fulfilling. Singer Shania Twain once famously said "I enjoyed working at McDonalds". Creating joy at work is about injecting passion into it and confronting rather than ignoring problems you see or the discomfort you feel.

In doing so you will either initiate the change you want to see or can walk away knowing that you tried.

**DON'T TANGO WHEN YOU WANT TO SAMBA**

You can improve your levels of joy and satisfaction at work by confronting the people and issues that are holding you back. Addressing dysfunctional systems, processes and procedures is part of this.

Don't be shy to become a solution provider. Your boss will likely thank you for it. Don't be afraid to notice the problem and solve it! Who knows, you may even create yourself a new job.

**THE TANGO**

In my early career, I had a successful job in sales. I loved my job! I worked 8am til 8pm Monday to Friday and on Saturdays too, but I didn't mind because I was fresh out of university, had a lovely office in London, was given the keys to a brand-new company car and was paid an enviable wage.

I enjoyed smashing sales targets and remained high on the leaders' board when the greats were cheered and every Friday at the head office in Mayfair.

We won champagne, raced supercars, enjoyed company ski trips and progressed through our Volkswagens to new BMW's and luxurious Porsches. Burnout was commonplace and staff turnover was high, but it was all good fun until it wasn't.

After a while, I'd had enough of using my day off purely to recuperate from the six-day working week, so I found a nine-to-five job elsewhere. However, before leaving, the Director and I had a chat about the way company property details were presented.

You see, managers who loved writing produced reams of details about each house for sale, waxed lyrical about its great selling points. Whereas managers who didn't enjoy writing produced property details that were concise and to the point.

Furthermore, reception rooms were called drawing rooms, lounges, sitting rooms and the like, so how were prospective customers or international clients to know they are all essentially the same thing? How were they to know they had been described using different words according to personal preference?

When all the details were collated on the central system and uploaded on-line for the world to see, property details were markedly different lengths. The was no uniformity, no branded company language and inconsistencies came to the fore.

**BY JOVE, SHE'S GOT IT!**

To cut a long story short, the company acknowledged that this was a significant issue with a potentially straightforward solution. I was requested to continue my role, with the added responsibility of training teams of photographers at the Head Office to become dual-expert professionals—property detail writers and photographers combined.

I was tasked with creating a company brand language and consistency across all London offices, producing training documentation and running workshops to roll out the new blueprint for presenting properties to the market globally.

Yet, at the age of 18, I was persuaded that doing a BSc in Business Management was the right thing to do. That rather painful journey, mostly through maths and economics (as well as other aspects I loved), culminated in a 2:1 degree. But it didn't float my boat.

## PROBLEM

My cohort joined investment banks, accountancy firms, or started their own businesses, while I felt somewhat stuck. So, I decided to work in a sales environment while figuring out the next steps in my life.

## PROPOSED SOLUTION

I met with my boss to say I was leaving and why, and because I spoke up, I was offered a new job as a trainer in the firm, and then another position in the marketing department and then in public relations. All 3 jobs involved a lot of writing; editing, copywriting, journalistic writing, managing people and more. I loved them all!

## THE RESULT – DANI'S NEW DANCE

I came full circle and returned to what I loved doing – creating marketing campaigns, investing in people, and growing businesses internationally.

After a few years, when I was ready to start a family, I founded a PR and Marketing business that allowed me to work from home. This quickly led to me becoming a resident expert in magazines, establishing Market Mall for Entrepreneurs, taking on the role of an Activator for The Great Outdoor Gym Company, and ultimately founding Stride Into Life and training to be a Health Coach.

Don't stay stuck doing the tango when your heart's desire is to samba. Walk your own path. Don't be afraid to try new things. Create the steps that bring you joy. Have fun dancing on others' dance floors but play your own music too. Move away from stressful work environments and towards those you feel passionate about. Don't settle.

## DO WHAT YOU LOVE! OUTSOURCE WHAT YOU DON'T.

Find out who you are and do a job you love as if your life depended on it, because it does!

Don't study engineering if you are a musician, or work as a gardener if you passionately want to bake, dance, or write. Explore opportunities in your current place of work before jumping ship or moving on.

If you are self-employed and detest doing your tax return, find a good local accountant and use the time you'd have spent on it to deliver more services and grow other income streams you love.

Question what other changes you can bring about to make your current job more enjoyable. Bruce Daisley, creator of the hit business podcast 'Eat Sleep Work Repeat' shares some great insights on how to create joy right where you are in his book 'The Joy of Work'.

He recommends we 'go for a walking meeting, shorten the working week, turn off notifications, go to lunch and have a digital sabbath' among other things. Such insights and changes can alter our perception of a job we think we dislike.

## REFLECT

Spend some time reflecting on how the journey of life has equipped you with additional skills and knowledge in your employment rather than seeing any stuck time as wasted time'. What did it teach you? How can you use it? My time in sales taught me how to grow my emotional intelligence and build rapport with thousands of customers.

Perhaps you feel stuck in a career you hate because you began in the wrong direction, then never got off that path. You can get off that path. The new path may not be perfect or straight, but it will likely be a path that sparks joy and provides more fulfilment. What does that path look like?

_____

_____

_____

_____

_____

_____

_____

_____

_____

_____

## TRUST YOURSELF – YOU KNOW THE WAY

Trust yourself as you begin to question, process, and find answers relating to which career fits you, and which job environment might suit you best.

In 2020, during lockdown, many of us discovered that working from home is the answer to our work/life balance and this alleviated the dysfunctional dances in our places of work.

Others discovered that having raised children; we didn't want to go back to teaching or administrative work. We wanted to work from home. We took up photography or personal training. We did another course or degree, or we explored other vocations.

We don't need a new baby or a pandemic to move us out of our stuck place at work. Instead, we can actively choose to become unstuck. We can ask good friends to be our soundboards, too, as their feedback can help facilitate this process. They know us well.

Good friends are often destiny helpers when it comes to our vocation – they are best placed to see our skills and giftings – and can honestly tell us the things we excel at and are not so good at.

Their honesty is a gift they can't give if we don't invite them to.

Find Joy in Work and say no to being stuck in stress, frustration, or burnout.

# STEP 18: Break Up with Fear Using Journalling
Fear teaches you a lot about yourself but you no longer need to be controlled by it

*"I learned that courage was not the absence of fear, but the triumph over it. The brave man is not he who does not feel afraid, but he who conquers that fear"*
*- Nelson Mandela*

**ANNA**

It was opening night and backstage, the atmosphere was electric. Anna had dreamed of opening a show her whole life but now the moment had arrived she felt sick.

*"I don't know what to do," Anna confided in Liv. "I'm not even on stage and my palms are sweating, my heart is racing, I feel like I'm going to faint. This is awful. What if they hate me tonight? What if they don't like the show?"*

*"When I feel like this my voice gets affected. I lost my words entirely once, don't you remember!?" Anna said.*

*"Anna" said Liv. "You are awesome. It's a brand-new show yes, but your last show was extended; the audience loves you! And here you are. This is your moment".*

*"What did you tell me on Friday?" smiled Liv. "You said that I am neither 'too much' or 'not enough' but that I am 'more than enough'. Ditto. So, I want you to enjoy every minute of this. You make us all fly Anna. Let this audience soar with you," Liv winked. "Now go, it's time. I'll see you on the other side. We love you!".*

# Step 18: BREAK UP WITH FEAR

W hat does the brave version of you need to tell Fear? Step 18 is to break up with the paralysing power of fear and tell Fear that it is no longer going to keep you stuck.

**Nothing happens to you; it happens for you**

All that has happened to you was an opportunity to grow – even in the most heinous circumstances. And there it is. The chance to 'move on' or remain 'stuck'. To 'overcome' or 'be overcome'.

In Step 18, we will begin with a creative process. There is no right or wrong way to approach this, but essentially, we will write a 'breakup letter' to Fear, outlining a better plan to combat paralysis, stress, insecurities, anxieties, and ill health. Additionally, we can express gratitude to Fear for the positive ways it keeps us safe. After all, without any fear, we could potentially put ourselves in harm's way.

Writing to Fear can be a really hard thing to do, so I've penned a 'break up' letter from myself to Fear to inspire and support you in this first step. Then we'll explore how journalling can help us stay free.

You may want to end your letter by wishing Fear all the best, and telling it that you are learning helpful ways to reflect, process and release fear.


*Dear Fear,*

*I'm writing to you from my heart to say you no longer have the power to control me. My relationship with you has been overwhelming at times and caused me to stay 'stuck' in my life.*

*Being sensitive to the desires, disapproval or anger of others made me follow paths and make decisions I didn't want to because I was afraid to make a mistake or lose the people or things I love.*

*You were the root of the decisions that controlled, coerced, and limited me. I am now prepared to lose every perceived comfort blanket to gain real life – I choose to be unstuck.*

## Step 18: BREAK UP WITH FEAR

*Getting approval fixes, being dominated, being controlled, or coerced by those around me felt frightening but strangely safe too. But it was not safe at all.*

*Fear, you have a lot to answer for - you caused me to minimise, deny or ignore my valid feelings like frustration, injustice, and pain. You boxed me in and caused a 'shutting down' in my life. I am no longer stuck with you and I'm stepping away from your manipulative persuasions.*

*I lived for approval in so many areas of my life, frightened to step off the tightrope in case my greatest fear of loss (both people or things) became a reality. I feared being abandoned. I believed if I stood up for myself or stood my ground I would be left behind, and that was a fear worse than death — not anymore, though.*

*You keep so many people stuck in 'fear of abandonment' but I am no longer one of them!*

*I'd rather be abandoned and free and alive, than attached to toxicity or fear.*

*Fear, you made me robotic. It felt safer to be seen and not heard. To withhold my thoughts and opinions from certain people for fear of the consequences. And to keep myself busy. Busy, busy. busy.*

*I felt wooden. The 'safe place' you implied I'd receive from you got me trapped being a 'human doing' not a 'human being'. I felt robotic and lifeless. I was shut down by you.*

*I am opening my life up because you caused me to live in a way that was 'expected of me' rather than 'enjoyed by me'.*

*Even now, I feel you rise up inside me. I'm scared to write this letter and show my vulnerability to whoever is reading this — but I, like so many others, am making wiser and more vulnerable choices these days. We choose, and I choose, freedom and authenticity over fear.*

*When I pursued healthy change in life, you chased me down with 'fear of the unknown,' but every time I was unsure, I chose to send you packing and to 'do it afraid'. This freed me from your clutches and I found peace, love and a quieter mind.*

*Thank you for helping me realise that the fear of staying stuck and not facing my demons, is worse than the fear of confronting them.*

*You wanted to give me counterfeit solutions of 'escape'. You told me to endure pain, hide trauma, maintain the status quo or run far from uncomfortable conversations.*

*You were wrong.*

*Fear, I lived so much of my childhood with FOMO (fear of missing out) and then as an adult I wanted affirmations from others as if my 'likeability' was in some way connected to the number of 'likes' I received.*

*Today I love myself enough not to need approval fixe' or be bound by how many 'likes' I get or don't get. I am not afraid of you. My affirmation comes from God and from those I choose to keep in my friendship circles.*

*I realise that you are responsible for so much dis-ease and disease in my life too. Do you know you make me and others physically ill, uncoordinated, unbalanced, inhibited and frozen? You give us stress, anxiety, digestive problems, headaches, itchy skin conditions, depression and ill health?*

*But no more - I don't need or want these gifts that just keep on giving thank you!*

*You are so noisy too. Once, you were the echo at home and the hum in my day. You have been very tiresome.*

*You encouraged me to garble and talk too much, to overstretch myself, and to avoid the places I planned to go to or things I wanted to do.*

*I don't live like that anymore. I live in the light these days, no longer in your shadow.*

*I want to thank you too though.*

*Thank you for warning me of dangers – for telling my mind, body and heart when things were not right. For alerting me when I could have burned myself on the hot pan or got into bad situations with unhealthy people. Sometimes I ignored you when you were trying to help me. I'm sorry for that. I'd like you to stick around only in the situations when you are helpful to me.*

*Thank you that fear of being not good enough helped me excel at school and in the workplace. I pushed myself way too much because of you, but thankfully I know how to manage myself better now.*

*Thank you for driving me to quiet places of withdrawal where I grew my gifts of writing, deep thinking, gaining knowledge and enjoying 'alone time' so what you meant for my harm and disconnection was used for good many times over. Thank you.*

*Thank you for showing me the toxic people, places and things I needed to step away from in my life. You used to really pressure and overwhelm me, causing me to make choices I was uncomfortable with or to cover up things that I should have shone light on, but you no longer control me in that way.*

*You are allowed in my life, at my table and as my friend in one capacity only – to help me 'notice' when things are not right or are downright dangerous. The dynamic of our relationship needed to change for a long while now.*

*My flaws make me human so I'm letting you know I'm aware I no longer need to fear anyone's opinion because I don't need to be perfect – for you or anyone else.*

*Fear, you made 'self-protection' such a high priority in my life. You taught me about, towing the line and walking a tight rope when I wanted to explore love and emotionally healthy spirituality.*

*I now know good leadership is not based on fear but on respect and kindness – and emotional intelligence.*

*I wish you well and will see you again on those occasions where your help is appreciated and needed; a hot oven, a toxic person, an invitation to overcome hard things. You are free to tell me when something is bad for me, painful or harmful to me, and for that I am grateful. But as for all the limiting stuff, I refuse to partner with it anymore.*

*All the best,*

*Dani x*

Take time to write your own letter to Fear and flow with whatever comes into your mind. If not today, then when? Let your mind and subconscious lead you and show you what to write. It doesn't have to be long but whatever you write will be powerful and life-changing. You are okay. You've got this!

_____
_____
_____
_____
_____
_____
_____
_____
_____
_____
_____
_____
_____
_____
_____
_____
_____
_____
_____
_____
_____
_____
_____

_____

_____

_____

_____

_____

_____

_____

_____

_____

_____

_____

_____

_____

_____

_____

_____

_____

_____

## TAKE UP JOURNALLING

Writing thoughts and feelings down is very healing and helps maintain optimal health on a daily basis. In just a few minutes each day, journalling is a way of reflecting on your progress in overcoming hard things and reflecting on your progress to wellness.

Did you know that 'journalist' comes from the word 'journal'?

Journalling allows us to explore, discover and process our thoughts and feelings on paper. It acts as a lasting record of how much we've grown and lets us see how far we've come. Where you've come from is as important as where you are going.

Neuroscience explains how 'writing things down' helps our wellbeing.

## WHY JOURNALLING IS GOOD FOR YOU

1) External storage – seeing our life journey journal in its location acts as a visual cue to remember to self-reflect and revisit our inner world regularly.

2) Encoding – when we write thoughts, feelings and ideas down, the things we perceive travel to the hippocampus in the brain where they are analysed. From there, decisions are made about what gets stored in long-term memory and what gets discarded. Writing improves the encoding process.

3) The Generation Effect - people can better memorise and retain information they generated themselves than material generated by others.

4) Authenticity - when we write down real thoughts and emotions, we also find ourselves thinking and living much less superficially.

5) Wellbeing - Research tells us that writing down thoughts and feelings helps us heal and overcome depression.

This was certainly the case for me. I suffered from post-natal depression after giving birth to 2 of my 3 children and writing, just a paragraph or so a day, really helped me to reflect, process and heal.

## DEPRESSION

I remember reading 'Depressive Illness, The Curse of the Strong' by Dr Tim Cantopher in that season and learning that people who develop depression '….usually want to put everything right, for everyone, including themselves, and are intolerant of symptoms, particularly anxiety or insomnia, which of course go hand in hand with stress and depression anyway'.

Dr Cantopher cites the problem of depression as 'the fear of fear'.

Perfectionists are prime candidates for depressive illness, wanting life to be perfect. 'If you spend your life worrying about the past, the future and your symptoms for long enough, eventually…. you will blow a fuse and develop a depressive illness.

---

*Unhappiness and stress come are rooted in spending too much time in self-recrimination from past perceived mistakes, and the fear of losses in the future*

---

Eckhart Tolle, the author of 'The Power of Now' dealt with his depression by giving up everything and living rough for a period, realising in the process that unhappiness and stress don't come from your circumstances or what happens to you in the now, but in spending too much time in self-recrimination for past perceived mistakes and fear of loss in the future.

Contemporary advice is sometimes to ignore the past but I have personally found that by facing the past and processing inner turmoil on paper rather than running away from it, I could feel it and so heal from it more deeply.

In 'Opening Up by Writing It Down, How Expressive Writing Improves Health and Eases Emotional Pain', Pennebaker and Smyth explain how after writing just a few sentences each day, people felt much more positive about themselves, their circumstances and the future.

I encourage you to buy yourself a journal and use it moving forward as your own 'self-development book' where you continue to be honest about your fears, thoughts, feelings and circumstances each day.

**MAXIMISE THE BENEFITS OF JOURNALLING**

### 1) Buy a journal that sparks joy in you.

Choose a colour that inspires or excites you and buy some nice stationary that you will enjoy using.

The sight of the journal will act as a visual cue for you to do something, which rather than feeling like a chore, will become a reward the more you use it. This is your new 'payoff'. The 'me time' is a new reward.

### 2) Clear a special space

Clutter clutters the mind. The special place you sit for 10 or 15 minutes a day should be your sacred space - clear of clutter and other distractions. So, mute your phone, clear away your laptop or tablet and create a special oasis space where your thoughts and feelings can flow. This process will become easier the more you practice.

### 3) Buy a candle or diffuser

Place a scent you love (a candle, or diffuser) in your special space. Neuroscience shows us that scent, emotion and memory are all intertwined. The journaling process becomes helpful and joyful, so it's useful to 'cement' this positive association in the brain using scent. As you smell the scent and journal, your nose knows, 'This is me-time, growth time, self-development time'. Fragrance creates such an immediate connection that brands like Nike are now using a signature scent (inspired in part by a soccer cleat in grass and soil) to create positive and memorable connections with their brand. What smell inspires you?

### 4) Choose a good time

Stay in your own lane and find a time that suits you when the house is not 'busy' and the distractions of everyday life, family, children, deliveries, and television are minimal. Remember, the more stillness you can create in the spacious place, the more you will hear what your body and mind are telling you.

### 5) Don't despise small beginnings

It's okay to start small and your own journalling process may only include a few words at first. You might be happier sketching your thoughts and feelings or using a combination of words, colours and pictures. Let it flow and don't be afraid to do whatever process is most meaningful to you.

### 6) Don't give up

You're making great progress by reading this book – you've already reached Step 18. Set a target for yourself to complete another three days in your journal, and then another three days, until you have a long chain of threes. If you miss a day, don't be too hard on yourself; just aim to continue your new healthy habit. Strive to create a chain of at least 21 days, as it typically takes 21 days to establish a new habit.

### 7) Write positive affirmations

Words are powerful. They are a creative force that transforms our environment and shape who we become. So jot down any positive affirmations that are particularly helpful to you. You can also speak them out. It may be something really simple like 'I am enough' or 'I am strong', or something more complex, 'I will no longer be seen and not heard' or 'I will be seen and heard because I have intrinsic value and what I have to say is important'.

I'm grateful to Patrick Mayfield, author of 'Leading Yourself: Succeeding from the Inside Out' who has also mentored me in recent years and helped me crystallise the reasons for and benefits of journalling.

**PART 6 ACTIVATIONS**

**PAY IT FORWARD - EMPOWER OTHERS**

**Step 16:**

Apologise to someone for mismanaging your emotions and tell them how you could and should have responded well to them, not reacted badly to them. Try again

**Step 17:**

Encourage a friend or colleague to find joy and value at work

**Step 18:**

Buy someone you care about a journal and encourage them to break up with Fear

# Step 18: BREAK UP WITH FEAR

# PART 7
# LET GO AND LAUGH

Well done for reaching Part 7. You've come a long way! The final steps empower us let go of anything still holding us back, and forgive ourselves and others. By now we feel grateful for the journey and are ready to let go of the past and boost our immune systems.

# Step 18: BREAK UP WITH FEAR

# STEP 19: Adopt an Attitude of Gratitude
## Gratitude is good for your health

*"The word gratitude is derived from the Latin word gratia, which means grace, graciousness, or gratefulness. It's a heartfelt thankful appreciation for what a person receives, whether its tangible or intangible"*
- Patrick Mayfield

**DANI**

*I'm thankful for health and healing this morning. I'm thankful for everything I've learned as a Health and Wellness Coach and for helping to bring my body's 11 systems into balance.*

*I'm grateful for lunch at The Veg Box Canterbury yesterday and for the Green smoothie bowl that nourished my digestive system. I'm thankful for the 100,000,000 neurons in my gut that send messages to my brain, and for the vagus nerve that allows communication to happen. Thank you for the wisdom of good principles. I'm grateful I know how to look after the microbiomes in my gut with delicious Saurkraut and Kimchi in my salads. Thank you for foods that help heal anxiety and depression.*

*Thank you for the Pilates classes that care for my lymphatic system and for the knowledge that, unlike my heart, my lymphatic system has no pump and needs me to move so that it can function properly. Movement is medicine. I'm so grateful to hear the waves this morning as I walked Poppy at the beach. The sky was beautiful!*

*I feel blessed to have seen the sunrise this morning and there's blossom on the apple tree in Cambridge (6th April). I'm grateful for the bees that pollinate our fruit trees and for the fruit they produce.*

*I'm processing big feelings this week, so I'm grateful for good friends who listen so well and love me. I'm thankful for opportunities to love others well too. Thank you for meaningful connections and life flow x*

# STEP 19: ADOPT AN ATTITUDE OF GRATITUDE

Gratitude refers to goodness in our lives and the source of the goodness. As the source usually lies at least partly outside of ourselves, gratitude and thankfulness help us connect to something larger than ourselves— whether to other people, God or nature.

Research shows us:

- Gratitude is strongly and consistently associated with greater happiness.
- Gratitude helps people feel more positive emotions, enjoy good experiences, improve their health, deal with adversity, and build strong relationships.

We can feel and express gratitude in many ways; we can apply it to the past (retrieving positive memories and being thankful for moments in childhood or past blessings), the present (not taking our life, people or things for granted), and the future (having a hopeful and optimistic outlook).

Like EQ (emotional intelligence), gratitude is a habit that we can always cultivate further.

As I explored the science behind the power of gratitude and started actively adopting it as a heart posture, I also found it very healing to start the day with gratitude. To really think about the past, present and future. What are you most grateful for right at this moment?

Even in the midst of trauma, grief or emotional pain of the past, we can be thankful for our narrative and that it gave us resilience and helps us understand and love others well. What will you be grateful for in the future? What skills do you have that are helping you to create the future your heart desires? That's a lot to be grateful for.

_____

_____

_____

_____

_____

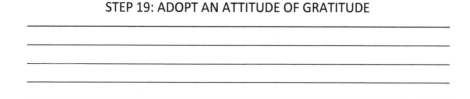

## WHAT DOES THE SCIENCE SAY?

Dr Martin Seligman at the University of Pennsylvania tested the impact of positive psychology interventions by asking his test subjects to write and personally deliver a letter of gratitude to someone who had never been properly thanked for their kindness.

Participants immediately exhibited a huge increase in happiness scores. This impact was greater than any other form of positive psychology intervention and the benefits lasted a month!

Studies have also shown how gratitude can improve relationships. Couples who take the time to express gratitude for their partners not only feel more positive toward them, as shown in the research, but also feel more at ease discussing concerns about their relationship.

This is exciting news for us because it indicates that our capacity to have courageous conversations with one another is supported by the power of gratitude. It appears that combining brave conversations (Step 4) with practicing gratitude (Step 19) will lead to revolutionary results.

With 280 million people in the world suffering from depression (The Priory), I'm encouraged by Dr Joshua Brown and Dr Joel Wong's research at the University of Indiana. They had a significant breakthrough in this area of mental health.

They studied nearly 300 adults, mostly college students, who were seeking mental health counselling at university for depression, anxiety and other related issues. Their findings were profound.

Brown and Wong randomly assigned their study participants into groups. Each was recruited just before they began their first session of counselling and on average, they reported clinically low levels of mental health at the time. Every group received counselling.

1) Group 1 wrote a letter of gratitude to someone each week for three weeks
2) Group 2 wrote about their deepest thoughts and feelings about negative experiences
3) Group 3 did not do any writing activity

Group 1 (the gratitude group) reported significantly better mental health four weeks and 12 weeks after their writing exercise had ended!

There are four key insights from this study that helped me personally:

**1. Gratitude unshackles us from toxic emotions**

Gratitude letter writing produces better mental health by shifting one's attention away from toxic emotions, such as resentment and envy. When you write about how grateful you are to others and how much other people have blessed your life, science shows it may become considerably harder to ruminate on negative experiences.

**2. Gratitude writing helps even if you don't share it**

Only 23 percent of participants who wrote gratitude letters sent them however, they still enjoyed the benefits of experiencing gratitude nonetheless.

So, if you're considering writing a thank-you letter to someone but are uncertain about whether to send it, I encourage you to write it anyway. The mere act of writing the letter can help you appreciate the people in your life and shift your focus away from negative and unhealthy feelings and thoughts.

**3. Gratitude's benefits take time**

The mental health benefits of gratitude writing in the study didn't emerge immediately but happened over time. Although the different groups in the study didn't differ in mental health levels one week after the end of the writing activities, the difference in mental health became more significant 12 weeks after the writing activities. This may be because letter writers discussed what they wrote with their counsellors or with others too.

So, when we begin our own journey of gratitude writing practise, we shouldn't be surprised if we don't feel dramatically better immediately after the writing. We can be patient and persevere knowing that the positive health benefits will materialise.

**4. Gratitude has lasting effects on the brain**

Three months after the psychology sessions began Brown and Wong discovered that the brains of the gratitude writers were processing information differently.

The gratitude letter writers showed greater activation in the medial prefrontal cortex when they experienced gratitude in the fMRI scanner. This effect was found 12 weeks after the letter writing began!

This indicates that simply expressing gratitude may have lasting effects on the brain, training the brain to be more sensitive to the experience of gratitude in the future, and resulting in improved mental health over time

**GRATITUDE IS SPIRITUAL AND REDUCES STRESS**

Talking to God (prayer), including being thankful to God and praying for others, is scientifically proven to reduce stress. And the good news is we can pray in any place, at any time and with anyone.

In his book '59 Seconds: Think a Little Change a Lot', Richard Wiseman shares research conducted by Neal Krause from the University of Michigan. He interviewed hundreds of people about the nature of their prayers, finances, and health.

Krause discovered that praying for self-seeking material things offers no protection to health and wellbeing but praying for others helps reduce the financial stresses and strains of the person doing the praying. So it's a lovely idea to start your day with prayers of thanks. 'Thank you for… (a person in your life). Focus on why you are grateful for them, and then pray for them.

**ENJOY JOURNALLING**

Gratitude is our superpower. So, we can look forward to journalling a gratitude list every day. It is medicine for the soul that has only positive side effects.

# STEP 19: ADOPT AN ATTITUDE OF GRATITUDE

## STEP 20: Forgive Yourself and Others
Actively choose free over stuck, through forgiveness

*"I really believe that when someone else does us harm, we're connected to that mistreatment like a chain. Because forgiveness is nothing less than an act of fidelity to an evil-combating campaign... Forgiveness is about being a freedom fighter"*
- Pastor Nadia Bolz-Weber

**HENRY**

*Henry battled with unforgiveness. Whilst he forgave motorists who cut him up or dented his car, there were things in life he just couldn't forgive. Namely, his mother's inexcusable lack of love towards him.*

*It caused him distressing self-harm and sleeplessness. It dented his pride and created bewilderment. How could he forgive this intolerable inner pain? Henry was flat-lining inside and anger's destructive force had taken over his life.*

> *"Forgiveness is easier said than done. It's one of the most difficult issues in life," his mentor Sally agreed. "Many of my clients find they need to forgive the same person daily, even after they've passed away. Why? Because unforgiveness can turn life into a prison of the mind Henry. The anger doesn't go away it just gets worse".*

> *"How might you be able to release some of your very valid pain this week Henry? Forgiveness doesn't mean what's happened is ok, but it protects your mind and body from unhelpful toxicity. You are free to choose. Emotional trauma and anger affect many of the body's systems and place a heavy load on the body as it works to maintain its default state of inner peace and balance" explained Sally.*

# STEP 20: FORGIVE YOURSELF AND OTHERS

I stumbled across Nadia's short video on forgiveness one day on YouTube and was blown away by it. Like many of us I wanted to know how to forgive others in a way that is real, deep, authentic, and healing. There's no doubt about it; unforgiveness makes us sick – it's like drinking poison and believing it will harm the person who hurt you. It won't.

Toxicity and being stuck is not something I want in my life so I was willing to 'fight' anything that brought those things to my doorstep. Arming myself with freedom meant disarming unforgiveness.

As Nadia eloquently says, "Maybe retaliation or holding onto anger about the harm done to me doesn't actually combat evil. Maybe it feeds it...So what if forgiveness is, rather than being like a pansy way of saying it's okay, actually a way of wielding bolt cutters and snapping a chain that links us."

Forgiveness is not about saying what happened to you is okay. It's about becoming unstuck and free. It's about not being controlled by the past. It's about landing a smack bang in the middle of 'life' and all the life you still have before you.

**FREE PEOPLE ARE POWERFUL PEOPLE**

Free people embrace the now rather than being stuck in the past

Free people find joy and laughter in their day

Free people see beauty in today rather than being tarnished by the ashes of what happened yesterday

Free people are not chained to bitterness or resentment.

Free people find warmth in their connection to life and to others

And all of this – this giant Stride into Life – is worth fighting for. It's worth forgiving for. It's worth moving out of the mud of unforgiveness, pain, disease and bitterness, and away from what happened to you.

Nadia concludes, "There really is a light that shines in the darkness, and the darkness cannot, will not, and shall not overcome it".

## REMOVE CONSTRICTION

Holding onto unforgiveness and harbouring bitterness or resentment is like walking around with boa constrictor snakes that keep biting us. Life's not the easiest when trying to navigate each day with snakes on our arms and legs! They have a tight grip on us, and limit our movements, our work, our connection with people, our happiness, and our peace.

As we ruminate and replay over and again what happened to us, the snakes bite us over and again, poisoning our hearts, minds and bodies with a cocktail of retaliation, retribution, unforgiveness, hatred and bitterness.

If we're not careful, we can even absorb so much of the venom (the worst of our enemy) we can, on some level, even start to become like them. Unforgiveness also makes us ill. The dis-ease we feel fills the mind, body and heart with aches, pains and symptoms synonymous with stress.

Instead, we can say, 'what you did was not okay but I refuse to be connected to it anymore,' and we can remove each boa constrictor.

## A HAPPIER, HEALTHIER YOU

Forgiveness improves our health and elevates mood, enhances optimism, guards against stress, and staves off anxiety and depression.

Some of us imagine that once we have forgiven someone, it's done and we're free (and that is sometimes the case), but for most of us, forgiveness is an ongoing choice that we need to make whenever unforgiveness rears its head.

## FORGIVENESS DOESN'T ALWAYS MEAN RECONCILIATION

Whether you have suffered shame, blame, rejection, betrayal, abuse or whatever happened to you, it's important to acknowledge that forgiveness doesn't mean reconciliation, although it might.

When we choose forgiveness and get unstuck, we don't need to return to the same relationship or accept the same damaging behaviours. You may, especially if abuse is involved, need to stand very firm against the offender's assumption that because you have forgiven them, things will continue where you left off.

In many cases, this is neither wise nor possible.

Rather we need to visit our inner world, set healthier boundaries and tell the other person what we need from them. Perhaps this is space or maybe we need to feel safe and reassured by them. We need them to demonstrate that they are committed to stopping their harmful or damaging behaviour.

Accountability is key. It's one thing to be told 'I won't do it again' and another to be shown accountable, demonstrative progress and accountable willingness to repair the tear(s).

Until you have seen someone's authentic and demonstrable willingness to change – often this means them attending counselling, doing a course or no longer surrounding themself by certain people, places or things – you will likely need to maintain distance from them.

**FORGIVENESS WHEN SORRY NEVER COMES**

Some of us feel stuck until the person who harmed us says sorry. Sometimes sorry never comes – what then? We rise above it and become even more badass.

When sorry never comes, we can recognise that all human beings are on their own journey and that people have varying levels of emotional intelligence (the ability to intelligently manage self and relationships with others well).

There may be a whole plethora of reasons why the person won't or can't say sorry to you (domestic abuse, addiction, special needs, lack of care, they passed away, low emotional intelligence, pride, their own pain, dysfunctional relationships, the list goes on....) but if we want to get unstuck, we can't let their 'stuff' keep us in chains.

Their stuff is theirs. I hope and pray they see the light and grow so that others don't suffer at their hands also, but in the meantime, my joy today is to focus on you.

Let them stay in their lane. And you stay in yours. Theirs may be 'cycles of the same'. But yours is '21 Steps to Unstuck' in this season.

## LOVE WINS

In my own journey to find inner peace and healing from dis-ease and disease, I was resourced by many leaders in their fields. This took the form of books, webinars, counselling, leadership courses, body chemistry analysis, freedom programmes, healthcare conferences, health coaching and medicine.

Each was invaluable; however, these resources could only take me so far. This is because *trauma is notoriously hard to heal* and 'unrelenting disappointment makes the heart sick' (Proverb).

Trauma is stored in the memory and emotional centres of the brain, such as the hippocampus and amygdala, so the body is activated when triggered by an event.

## DON'T SETTLE FOR 'ALMOST HEALED'

For me, the difference between 'almost healed' and 'healed' was letting God's love in; accepting that I'm the apple of his eye no matter what (as are you) and choosing to believe that Jesus can and does heal the broken hearted.

I came to the realisation that we simply don't need to carry the heavy weight of needing acknowledgement or apologies from those that cause harm in order to feel okay. They may be unwilling to offer either. We can all choose to live and create a beautiful life.

I learned to love myself, and to hand the people, places and things that hurt me over to God. Why? Bitterness, hurt and anger cloud our judgement. But God is more than able to deal with whatever happened – after all, he never sleeps and knows it all. This is no cop out. This is doing all you can to get unstuck, and leaving what you can't do to God.

I believe when we reconceptualise any injustice in this way, we say yes to complete wholeness and freedom. We realise His job is 'righteous judge' and ours is to 'love ourselves and others well'.

We can't do that through a filter of bitterness or bewilderment. *Love wins* means stepping away from toxicity and embracing love; a deeper, purer love. Love for self. And love for others.

Perhaps the most famous Bible verse is 'God is love'. So, when I'm running on empty in life, I place my trust in this truth and go to the source of love itself. To me, that's priceless, powerful and utterly beautiful.

# STEP 20: FORGIVE YOURSELF AND OTHERS

# STEP 21: Embrace the Science of Joy and Laughter
## Choose joy to boost your immune system

*'Laughing will lift your mood, reduce stress, make you healthier, help you bond with people and activate the empathy system in the brain. Let's choose to laugh more!'*
- Dr Caroline Leaf

**ISAAC**

*It was a bright sunny day in Croydon and Clio had popped in to visit her new neighbour Bayo and his family.*

"Isaac means 'to laugh,'" chuckled Bayo as he looked at his 5-year-old singing Pharrell Williams' 'Happy'.  And my own name has African origins and means 'the crown meets joy".

"We actually found 50 baby names that mean joy or laughter. Would you believe it? Lettie, Abigail, Joy, Laticia, Annabelle, Hasvi, Hani, Gili, Ron... That last one was made popular by J.K. Rowling. But we liked 'Isaac'".

"He's joyful by name, joyful by nature. He grows more handsome every day! My friend, it's less 'hip hop' and more 'hip hip hooray' in our home every day" Bayo chortled.  "The more we choose to laugh, the better we feel. No matter what, a deep belly laugh is medicine for the mind, body and soul".

# STEP 21: EMBRACE THE SCIENCE OF JOY AND LAUGHTER

Children laugh up to 500 times a day, whereas adults laugh just 3 - 5 times a day. Research consistently proves that love, laughter and hope can help the body fend off disease. So, with such low levels of laughter in adults, how is this negatively affecting our health?

Laughter is an icebreaker and a stress buster with lasting benefits beyond the moment. Laughter is also a natural pain reliever (it's the wisdom behind laughing gas).

**JOY TRULY IS MEDICINE**

According to professional Joy Activist and speaker Sue Jameson, just one positive event boosts the immune system for 2 days.

Sue reveals how studies worldwide show proven benefits of laughter, including:

- Exercising of the cardiovascular system
- Stimulation of T-cells in our immune system (just 1 positive event boosts the immune system for 2 days)
- Reduction of cholesterol and blood sugar
- Improvement in stress resistance
- Control of blood pressure
- Improvement in circulation
- Easing of abdominal disorders

Laughter tells the body to release a flood of natural painkillers called endorphins which are also released by physical exercise.

*** Sue introduced me to the profound story of Norman Cousins, who you may have heard of. Born in 1915, he is sometimes called 'the Father of Laughter Therapy' and used the power of laughter to heal (after being diagnosed with ankylosing spondylitis, an intensely painful form of arthritis).

Norman chose to tackle his illness by setting up a movie projector in his hospital room and watching comedies and classic episodes of Candid Camera. In between episodes, he chose to stay upbeat and relaxed. He discovered that 10 minutes of deep belly laughing would give him 2 hours of pain-free sleep with no pain relief medication.

Within months, he not only regained motion in his joints but felt the pain disappear. He made a near full recovery from his supposedly "incurable" disease, having been given in 1 in 500 chance of making a recovery. You can read more about his journey in his book 'The Anatomy of an Illness'.

**What other effects does humour have on our body?**

More recently, Researchers at Loma Linda University School of Medicine found that people who watched a comical 1 hr long video experienced a significant drop in the stress hormones cortisol and adrenaline. These hormones contribute to a wide range of illnesses, including heart disease and depression.

I was also excited to hear about a discovery by scientists in Baltimore back in 2005. They discovered that laughter might be tied to the healthy function of blood vessels, appearing to cause the tissue in the inner lining of our blood vessels to dilate in order to increase blood flow.

They discovered that people with heart disease were 40 percent less likely to laugh in a variety of situations compared to people of the same age without heart disease.

Just think, laughing can reduce the risk of cardiovascular disease!

If laughter is so good for us, why are we not doing it more, and why do we condition the laughter out of children?

There is so much evidence to support the health benefits of laughter, joy and gratitude we can afford to question why we tell our children to 'be quiet' and 'stop being silly' when they are goofing around and having fun!

It's clear that embracing gratitude, laughter, joy and love are keys to turning the tide on sickness and ill health. Could generations of your family suffering from stress, depression and anxiety become a thing of the past? Will you be the joy activist and freedom fighter who changes the habits of a lifetime in your home and normalises laughter for happiness and health? How could you do this in your home?

_____

_____

_____

_____

_____

_____

_____

_____

_____

_____

## JOY AND LAUGHTER AT WORK

### There are plenty of reasons to laugh a lot in the workplace too

"A decade of research proves that happiness raises nearly every business and educational outcome: raising sales by 37%, productivity by 31%, and accuracy on tasks by 19%, as well as a myriad of health and quality of life improvements" Harvard Business Review – Shawn Achor, The Happiness Advantage.

Joy and laughter can also be used at work to enhance team building and wellness. Sue Jameson explains that the benefits include:

- Encouraging efficiency and productivity
- Motivating staff
- Enhancing communication skills
- Improving leadership
- Cultivating innovation and creativity
- Developing problem-solving skills
- Increasing attention span
- Reducing absenteeism
- Creating positive work environments

## STEP 21: EMBRACE THE SCIENCE OF JOY AND LAUGHTER

**ENJOY LIFE**

Businesses across the world are actively promoting joy and the enjoyment of work.

A few years ago I was invited to interview Kay Chaston, the CEO of Enjoy-Work at Chiswick Park in London, and I was intrigued. Enjoy-Work, as the name says, is a unique work environment designed with one thing in mind – enjoyment at work – and it has seen phenomenal success as Kay explained to me.

'Chiswick Park is home to some of the world's leading companies and thousands of people, with its all-pervasive belief that if people enjoy work, they do better work – if they do better work, you have a better business'.

Corporations are referred to as guests and include the headquarters of Starbucks, Vue International, Swarovski and Pokémon. Having worked in Chiswick Park myself, I concur with the benefits of joy and laughter at work. Absolutely everything there was designed to have a positive impact on people's health and wellbeing. The very landscaping (coupled with innovative experiences of daily joy, fun, and laughter) had a hugely positive impact on my working day.

Whilst Enjoy-Work used to look like lakes with bikes to cycle around on, a beautiful bloom or chocolate placed on my desk, and fun events at lunchtimes, today Enjoy-Work Healthcare has taken things to another level and does even more, providing Wellbeing Seminars and Health Screening, an on-site physio and intravenous vitamins.

Wellness, joy and laughter are the future of our workplaces and wellbeing. And they are the final step to being unstuck at home and at work.

\*\*\* Take some time to reflect on how laughter and joy could help alleviate any health symptoms you may be experiencing. What would the impact be on your home life and work life, if you chose to laugh more?

What could you laugh at today that you might normally feel stressed or irritated by?

**PART 7 ACTIVATIONS**

**PAY IT FORWARD – EMPOWER OTHERS**

**Step 19:**

Encourage someone in your family to write a thank you letter and explain the benefits of gratitude.

**Step 20:**

Explain the healing power of forgiveness to a friend who is hurting and struggling to 'let it go.'

**Step 21:**

Put on a funny movie and enjoy deep belly laughing with your friends or family.

# HOST OR JOIN A 21 STEPS TO UNSTUCK LIFESTYLE BOOK GROUP

## The 21 Steps to unstuck leads to a healthier, happier life

*The 21 Steps to Unstuck is not a book to be read once and put down. It is one that should be by our side and read continuously to refine how we deal with issues continuously through our lives*
*- Dr John Bolodeoku, JB Consulting MDP, UK*

**Join a 21 Steps to Unstuck Lifestyle Book Group**

If you want to continue overcoming, and practice what you've learned, start or join a 21 Steps to Unstuck Lifestyle Group. You can email Dani@strideintolife.com to register as a host, and all in person and Zoom groups will be updated at Strideintolife.com.

Sharing your journey with others who seek to improve their quality of life is a great way to activate healing from dis-ease and disease. Each person in the group can feel authentic and known, loved, valued and accepted.

Your group could be a corporate or healthcare group, a religious or community group, a home group, a friends or family group, or a follow-on group. Follow-on groups can work well after other courses like the Freedom Programme.

Connection in small groups activates positive change and healing, transforming outcomes in families, friendships, workplaces, social circles and communities.

**Start Your Own Group Using the Book**

Sharing the insights in the 21 Steps with others is simple. You don't need to be experienced in leading a group, and it can be rewarding to run it together with a colleague, friend or family member.

Simply set aside 21 topic sessions (or 11 longer sessions) and follow the progressive steps, activations and discussion points in the book.

It's recommended to cover 1 Step each session, giving enough time and space for people to share, grow, connect and build relationally.

## What Happens in the Group?

Groups use the book as a progressive map. They share good news, struggles and experiences, encourage one another, create meaningful connections, practice active listening and share experiences of emotional or physical healing.

Group discussion, connection and reflection provides a wider perspective than the exciting transformation of your own personal journey. Others will no doubt love to hear how the steps are changing your life.

## Transforming Lives Together

As a Lifestyle Book Group leader in the past, I found our common bond made us healthier. We became stronger together. We developed deep friendships through our shared experiences. We learned new ideas about wholeness, purpose, and living free. We became the best versions of ourselves, together.

## Camaraderie and Common Goals

In the field of wellness, my goal is always for people to leave feeling more open, whole, relaxed and joyful. The goal of group sessions is no different. In groups people find camaraderie. They become more open, loving and compassionate. This in itself, reduces stress and feelings of dis-ease, isolation or anxiety. Making your feelings known to yourself and others is life-giving.

## Pursue Health and Wholeness Together

Health comes from a root word meaning 'to make whole'. To live in optimal wellness. If not today, then when? If not you, then who? Loving yourself and others means loving well, loving from inside yourself and loving beyond yourself. Giving and receiving love is very healing.

## Increase Your Motivation and Commitment to Host or Join a Group

Science proves that a person must feel *motivated and committed* in order to follow through on a goal. So, the following questions help ensure your worthy goal to start a Group is achievable. What kind of Group you'd most feel motivated and committed to start or join?

## Finding Your Members

- Who may be ready and wanting to start this journey with you?
- Who in your family might benefit from this?
- Who is your current social network?
- Will this be a home group?
- Could this group work well in a corporate setting or as a healthcare or teambuilding programme?
- Could your local bookshop support you with their venue or to reach people who'd be interested? Many run book groups.
- Could your local religious or community centre help support you with a venue or to reach their members who might be interested?
- Which local charity might you be able to support by hosting this group for their members?
- Will you use word of mouth or social media to spread the word?
- Will it be an open or closed group?
- How many people will be in it? I recommend a maximum of 8.
- How often will the group meet?
- Will you integrate other activities as part of your group, like a walk, a meal or other events?
- Will you meet face to face or virtually?

Group leaders receive regular support and connection with me, Dani Simpson. You'll find more information at Strideintolife.

## How to Start and End the Group Session

1) Welcome and check-in. Ask everyone to say 2 words describing how they are feeling today, for example 'excited but overwhelmed' or 'tired and optimistic'. This breaks the ice and gives permission for people to be real and authentic.

2) Remind everyone that the group is a confidential space where nothing shared leaves the space unless there is a safeguarding issue. Basic safeguarding courses are available online for just a few pounds and are invaluable regardless. Safeguarding is our collective responsibility as fellow citizens.

3) Take turns to read and lead. Sharing roles helps people feel more empowered, motivated, committed to and invested in the group. It will become clear as the weeks unfold how each group wants to organise itself, so don't worry at the beginning.

4) Gently notice if anyone is not participating and ask them if they'd like to read or have anything to share, explaining that there is no pressure at all to do so but they are welcome to.

5) Practice active listening with empathy, curiosity, care and compassion.

6) Acknowledge what others are saying. Affirm people with encouragement and eye contact while they are sharing.

7) Resist the temptation to give unsolicited advice to others. Let everyone stay in their own lane and you in yours. Find joy in journeying together.

8) End the session with a checkout and what's next? Ask everyone to say 2 words describing how they are feeling now and what they are going to do next. For example, "I'm feeling energised but fearful. I'm going to mow the lawn now". The session has finished. Thank everyone for coming.

Visit Strideintolife.com for more information and I look forward to hearing about your wellness journey.

# SUBSCRIBE TO HEALTHIER, HAPPIER HOMES, WORKPLACES AND COMMUNITIES

Thank you for travelling 21 Steps with me. It's been a pleasure to share my journey with you.

If you enjoyed this book then you might like to **subscribe** to my free newsletter. Doing so means you'll also be the first to hear about my other writing, group programmes, coaching sessions and projects. I enjoy recommending the best books I'm reading, as well as fresh insights, and programmes run by other organisations and charities that you might find helpful. I've included some at the end of this book.

**You can sign up at Strideintolife.com**

### *PARENTS AND SCHOOLS*

The transformative tools, ideas and strategies from *The 21 Steps to Unstuck* can be applied broadly to all ages and stages of life so you'll find plenty of useful behavioural change concepts in the book. However, I'm rolling out a programme developed specifically for parents and schools; the *Worry to Wellness* programme will be widely available from 2024.

**You can sign up at Strideintolife.com**

### BUSINESSES

I've heard from business leaders, entrepreneurs and start-ups about how the *The 21 Steps to Unstuck* can help run better businesses. Progressive leaders want outstanding support that empowers employees to excel, be more effective and live in optimal wellness.  Rather than paying 'lip service' exercise, health and wellbeing are increasingly valued for reduced absenteeism, increased productivity, improved succession planning and optimal employee engagement. Business specific content is being developed in partnership with a London Business School.

**You can sign up at Strideintolife.com**

# FURTHER READING AND RESOURCES

The Joy of Work, Bruce Daisley

Eat, Sleep, Work, Repeat, Bruce Daisley

Leading Yourself: Succeeding from the Inside Out, Patrick Mayfield

Caring Enough to Confront, David Augsburger

Women who Love Too Much, Robin Norwood

Depressive Illness: The Curse of the Strong, Tim Cantopher

Cleaning up Your Mental Mess, Dr. Caroline Leaf

Spoon Fed: Why Almost Everything We've Been Told About Food is Wrong, Tim Spector

Rushing Women's Syndrome: The Impact of a Never-Ending To-Do List and How to Stay Healthy in Today's Busy World, Dr Libby Weaver

Atomic Habits: Tiny Changes Remarkable Results, Tim Clear

Running on Empty; Overcome your Childhood Emotional Neglect, Jonice Webb PhD

Emotional Intelligence and Social Intelligence: The New Science of Human Relationships, Dr Daniel Goleman, Ph.D.

Permission to Feel, Prof Marc Brackett

The Highly Sensitive Person: How to Survive and Thrive When the World Overwhelms You, Dr Elaine N. Aron. Ph.D.

59 Seconds: Think a Little Change a Lot, Richard Wiseman

Think and Eat Yourself Smart, Dr Caroline Leaf

Keep Your Love On, Danny Silk

The Power of Vulnerability: Teachings on Authenticity, Connection and Courage, Brené Brown

The Anatomy of an Illness as Perceived by the Patient, Normal Cousins

Emotionally Healthy Spirituality, Peter Scazzearo

Living with the Dominator, Pat Craven

Narcissism Exposed, Patricia King

The Sociopath Next Door, Martha Stout PhD

Enjoy-work.com

Mind.org.uk

Thefreedomprogramme.co.uk

Womensaid.org.uk

Restored-uk.org

Restoredlives.org

Thirtyoneeight.org

Relate.org.uk

Joy-activist.com

(Free laughter CD download: www.joy-activist.com/immunoboost)

Patrickmayfield.com

Enjoy-work.com

Healthcoachesacademy.com

Drindra.co.uk

# BIBLIOGRAPHY

P31 Crime Survey for England and Wales CSEW, crime survey.co.uk

p36 Switch On Your Brain: the Key to Peak Happiness, Thinking and Health, Dr Caroline Leaf

p41 Patrick Holford, CEO of the Food for the Brain Foundation, is widely recognised as Britain's leading spokesman on nutrition and mental health issues.

p43 National Institute for Health and Clinical Excellence, 2022.Nice.org.uk

p50 Social buffering; relief from stress and anxiety, Takefumi Kikusui, James T Winslow and Yuji Mori, 2006 The Royal Society, Ncbi.nlm.nih.gov

p53 World Health Organisation, 2019, health topics, noncommunicable diseases, Who.int

p54 Human Rights. The United Nations, Un.org

p52 Romans chapter 12 verse 2, New International Version 'Do not conform to the pattern of this world, but be transformed by the renewing of your mind.

P81 Domestic Abuse Bill, 3 March 2020, The Home Office

P81 Tackling Violence Against Women and Girls Strategy, 21 July 2021, the Home Office

P99 Rayramoscoaching@gmail.com

P99 TED talk, The Power of Vulnerability, Dr Brené Brown

p117 Psychosomatic Medicine Journal: Loneliness, Social Isolation, and Living Alone Associations with Mortality Risk in Individuals Living with Cardiovascular Disease, January 2023

p126 The Drama Triangle, Eric Burns, Fairy Tales and Script Drama Analysis, 1968

p128 The Winners Pyramid, Acey Choy, 1990

p184 280,000,000 in the world have depression, Priorygroup.com

p200 University of Maryland Medical Centre Study, Baltimore, March 19, 2005 'Laughter helps blood vessels function better.'

P201 Happiness isn't the result of success; it's the cause of it. Shawn Achor, The Happiness Advantage

# CREATING A WORLD IN THE WELLNESS ZONE

The Zone of Dis-ease is a pathway to the Zone of Disease. Actively choose wellness for optimal emotional, spiritual and physical health

*"Your energy flows where your focus goes"* - Dr Indra Barathan

| Zone of Disease | Zone of Dis-ease | *Zone of Wellness* |
|---|---|---|
| Depression | Emotional pain | *Energy* |
| Exhaustion | State of 'alert' | *Joy* |
| Chronic skin issues | Nerves | *Vitality* |
| Medications | Headaches | *Peace* |
| Heart disease | Dry skin | *Forgiveness* |
| Overwhelm | Digestive problems | *Connection* |
| Fibromyalgia | I just need to…. | *Love* |
| Issues of the gut | Poor sleep | *Gratitude* |
| Feeling terrible | I'm 'not too bad' | *Feeling great* |
| Life-less-ness | Life is pretty stressful | *Life is healthy* |

*We are created for wellness. So, despite what happened, regardless of hard things and no matter the multiple diagnoses, my innate healing came from aligning myself with the Zone of Wellness and giving my body permission to follow suit.*

*I'm no medical Doctor, but for me, the 21 Steps to Unstuck created a new way of life. Choosing wellness allowed dis-ease and disease to gradually leave. It never wanted to be there in the first place. I transitioned to the Zone of Wellness and my desire is for you to find yours too; your place of balance and health.*

*Today I'm medication free but much more than that I have a spring of life. In the Zone of Wellness, our love for humanity and for life itself overwhelms everything that feels overwhelming. God bless you.*

Milton Keynes UK
Ingram Content Group UK Ltd.
UKHW020630150923
428734UK00015B/283